African American Bioethics

African American Bioethics
Culture, Race, and Identity

Lawrence J. Prograis Jr.
Edmund D. Pellegrino
Editors

Georgetown University Press/Washington, D.C.

As of January 1, 2007, 13-digit ISBN numbers have replaced the 10-digit system.

13-digit
Paperback: 978-1-58901-164-9
Cloth: 978-1-58901-163-2

10-digit
Paperback: 1-58901-164-3
Cloth: 1-58901-163-5

Library of Congress Cataloging-in-Publication Data

Symposium on African American Perspectives in Bioethics (2004 : Georgetown University)
    African American bioethics : culture, race, and identity / Lawrence J. Prograis, Jr., and Edmund D. Pellegrino, editors.
    p. ; cm.
"Conference held on September 23–24, 2004 at Georgetown University titled Symposium on African American Perspectives in Bioethics and Second Annual Conference on Health Disparities"—Pref.
    Includes bibliographical references and index.
    ISBN-13: 978-1-58901-163-2 (hardcover : alk. paper)
    ISBN-10: 1-58901-163-5 (hardcover : alk. paper)
    ISBN-13: 978-1-58901-164-9 (pbk. : alk. paper)
    ISBN-10: 1-58901-164-3 (pbk. : alk. paper)
    1. Medical ethics—Congresses. 2. African American philosophy—Congresses. 3. Health services accessibility—United States—Congresses. I. Prograis, Lawrence. II. Pellegrino, Edmund D., 1920- III. Conference on Health Disparities (2nd : 2004 : Georgetown University) IV. Title.
    [DNLM: 1. African Americans—United States—Congresses. 2. Bioethical Issues—United States—Congresses. 3. Cross-Cultural Comparison—United States—Congresses. 4. Health Services Accessibility—ethics—United States—Congresses. WB 60 S989a 2007]
    R724.S937 2004
    174'.957—dc22

                                                            2006031183

⊗ This book is printed on acid-free paper meeting the requirements of the American National Standard for Permanence in Paper for Printed Library Materials.

14   13   12   11   10   09   08   07   9   8   7   6   5   4   3   2
First printing

Printed in the United States of America

This volume is gratefully dedicated to Marian Secundy and Harley Flack, through whose work and example the whole of bioethics has become better sensitized to the importance of a cultural perspective in ethics decisions.

CONTENTS

Acknowledgments

The editors are deeply indebted to the contributors of this volume, for without their participation and sharing of their "epistemic stance" and "internal perspective," there would be no *African American Bioethics: Culture, Race, and Identity*. The development of this volume arose through conversations between the editors about the conference and book titled *African American Perspectives on Biomedical Ethics* held more than fifteen years ago. This led to the development of another conference titled "Symposium on African American Perspectives in Bioethics and Second Annual Conference on Health Disparities," held on September 23–24, 2004, at Georgetown University. The conference was sponsored by the University of the District of Columbia and the Lombardi Comprehensive Cancer Center, Georgetown University; Minority Partnership Program, the Center for Clinical Bioethics, Georgetown University; and the Office of Research on Women's Health, National Institutes of Health. This conference and the present book would not have been possible without their financial and other support.

We want to acknowledge and thank Ms. Marti Patchell, whose administrative support was instrumental to the success of the conference and this book. We would also like to extend our thanks to Ms. Chloe Anne Free, Dr. Peter Shields, Ms. Donelle O'Meara, and Ms. Regina Jackson for their support with the conference and the book.

Finally, we would like to acknowledge the continued and unwavering support of our families and friends. It is your encouragement and support that has led to the completion of this volume.

INTRODUCTION

Culture and Bioethics: Where Ethics and Mores Meet

Edmund D. Pellegrino

"CULTURE" is perhaps the slipperiest concept in the social sciences.[1] Some years ago, Kroeber and Kluckhohn collected 164 definitions.[2] Of the many definitions available, we believe Kuper best captures the connotations of the word in his crisp characterization of culture as a "collective cast of mind."[3]

In this book we have taken a "collective cast of mind" to be a summation of all those things that give identity to persons, nations, ethnic groups, and organizations. Under this rubric we include all those things humans value, those things that define them as who they are, what they perceive themselves to be and want to be. These are the things they value enough to work for, live for, and die for. These are things that define their view of the good life and shape their morals, that is, their judgments of right and wrong, good and evil.

Every human and every group has its own perception of a specific configuration of values and beliefs that reflects its history, life experiences, and aspirations. Humans belong to many "cultures" in this sense: to a nation, family, club, political party, and so on. No two persons have precisely the same "cast of mind" as the others who share their "culture." However, it is in those things that are held in common that the profile of a culture is established.

African Americans, therefore, like all Americans, have a collective cast of mind on some things and individualized perspectives on many others. The essays in this collection indicate that two experiences in the lives of black Americans in the United States seem to be shared in common. One is the experience of color discrimination, the scars of slavery, and the depreciation of black people as human beings by the dominant culture. The other is the collective memory of their African roots, with its many unique cultures and customs transmitted from previous generations.

Certain features of these two experiences are shared and produce the "epistemological stance" about which J. L. A. Garcia writes in chapter 1. As the individual accounts of the essayists attest, African Americans as individuals weight these experiences sometimes differently in their own lives. So, while there is a collective cast of mind, it must not be interpreted as a stereotype lest it become a caricature to those who have not had the same experiences.

Included in any cast of mind is the intersection and tensions between customs and practices, between their mores and the rational justification for those practices, that is, their ethics. Recently and belatedly, bioethicists have begun to recognize this fact. Social scientists and humanists have urged that socioeconomic, political, and historical realities must be taken into account in bioethics.[4] Now the question for bioethicists is to discern how much weight should be given to each individual's and each group's customs and practices.

Evolution of Bioethics

Modern bioethics is barely thirty-five years old. It grew out of a 2,500-year tradition of medical ethics. Little or no formal justification of these ancient norms from a small group of Greek physicians took place until the late 1960s and early 1970s. Then theologians and philosophers undertook a critical and formal analysis of received norms and of new challenges to those norms. In the 1980s, humanists and social scientists expanded our understandings of the moral life. Bioethics became an interdisciplinary enterprise, which it is still today.

One result of the multidisciplinary approach has been a much richer comprehension of the complexities of moral decision and accountability.[5] Another result is exposure of the tensions that can arise between the ways social sciences and the ways philosophy and theology view moral problems and issues.[6]

Moral philosophers have generally focused on universal principles and norms based on a common human nature shared by all humans. Social scientists have focused on particular expressions of these norms with heavy reliance on descriptive and empirical studies. A conceptual question for bioethics in the years ahead is how to accommodate these two approaches and take advantage of each without one capitulating to the other.

This tension surfaces when cultural beliefs about right and good come into conflict with the more generally promulgated ethical norms of bioethics. How is priority to be established between the cultural definition of a moral norm and the critical definition of that norm by formal ethics? How do we respect cultural diversity without granting ethical hegemony to every cultural belief? Are the normative perspectives of moral philosophy and "culture" incommensurable, or do they complement and supplement each other?

Background of This Volume

It was against this background of transformations in bioethics that, more than fifteen years ago, our first conference on African American perspectives in bioethics was convened.[7] Three Howard University faculty members— Drs. Marian Secundy, Robert Murray, and Harley Flack—and I asked ourselves several questions about African American experiences with bioethics. Was there a distinctively African American cultural perspective(s) on bioethics? In what did it consist? How did it become expressed in health care decisions? What were its moral roots in the African American experience in America and in Africa?

These questions arose in each of our own teaching experiences with African American students of the health professions and in our clinical contacts with African American patients. Empirical data were scanty. Many, though not all, African Americans seemed to share perspectives at variance with the values and norms then shaping academic bioethics. These variances were most often manifest in decisions about the conduct of the end of life, organ donation, patient autonomy, participation in clinical research studies, patient-physician relationships, and the place of religion and folk medicine in clinical care. In a more general way, there was a distrust of the notion of bioethics itself and its role if any in personal decisions.

We sought a better grasp of the moral and ethical roots of these differences as they were perceived by African Americans. We hoped too to encourage African Americans to enter the field of bioethics. To these ends, we convened a group of African American scholars to consider our questions and other questions they might deem appropriate. These scholars asked us to invite white commentators so that there might be an intercultural dialogue on the issues as well.

In the essays that emerged from the first conference there was general agreement that African Americans, and Africans as well, did have moral beliefs and values that diverged from the Western and Anglo-American values that dominated academic bioethics. These beliefs had their roots in the uniqueness of the African American experience: in some of the traditions of African culture, and especially in the experience of slavery, and the residual discrimination that is still an actuality in American life.

Development of the Current Volume

A few years ago, Dr. Lawrence Prograis, then deputy director for the Division of Allergy, Immunology and Transplantation, National Institute of Allergy and Infectious Diseases, National Institutes of Health (NIH), joined the Center for Clinical Bioethics as a Fellow and Visiting Scholar. Dr. Prograis was deeply concerned about the conceptual foundations for an African American perspective. As clinicians, Dr. Prograis and I revisited the questions addressed by the first conference and wondered if the passage of a decade would result in a change in perspective. We invited African American scholars to consider the issues. Some had participated in the first volume, some had not. This occasioned the present group of essays.

Much had transpired in the intervening decade in bioethics. Some bioethicists, far too belatedly in the opinion of social scientists, had begun to appreciate the place of culture in bioethical decisions. Bioethics itself had expanded rapidly to become a world movement. Most countries in the developed world were establishing their own research and teaching centers in bioethics. In the process, Anglo-American ethical norms, and particularly those of principlism, were subjected to critical examination, often from a different cultural perspective.

At the same time, bioethics was becoming a subject of sociopolitical concern. On the international level, the moral significance of the UN Declaration on Human Rights, with its emphasis on human dignity, provided a stimulus. The World Health Organization formulated norms for the conduct of human experimentation. The World Medical Association, the Council of Europe, and the United Nations Educational, Scientific and Cultural Organization (UNESCO) each worked on declarations of norms for professional ethics and bioethics. International, intercultural, and interdisciplinary conferences have become commonplace.

During this period, the number of African American bioethicists has grown, though not very rapidly. Tuskegee University established a Center for Bioethics under the directorship of Marian Secundy, one of the conveners of our first conference. African Americans who had achieved prominence in law, medicine, and the social sciences raised questions from within the establishment of bioethics. Cultural anthropologists continued their emphasis on the ineradicability of cultural belief in ethical decisions—not just among African Americans but also among the multitudinous cultures of the new wave of immigrants to America. The bioethical implications of culture on a global scale were just beginning to be examined.[8]

It is now clear that the changing demography of America requires that practitioners and students of all the health professions develop cultural competence and communication skills.[9] Emphasis on empirical studies is requisite concomitantly if cultural competence is not to be based on caricatures and stereotypes. The lessons to be learned from the African American experiences with bioethics are analogous to those of a large segment of new Americans.

It is against this changing backdrop that the essays in this second volume should be interpreted. While much has changed so far as the African American experience goes, there has not been fundamental change in the perceptions of the scholars we convened. On the whole, they agree that there is an African American perspective and that it has been shaped by the unique history of black people in America.

This "stance," as J. L. A. Garcia sees it, and the other essayists reaffirm in a variety of different ways, shapes the topics, methods, and moral claims of African Americans today. It accounts for the mistrust of many African Americans for organizations, health professionals, clinical investigators, and administrators. Garcia is frank to say that, given the negative aspects of their experience, African Americans should be antimajoritarian, antiutilitarian, antiscientific, and antisituationist and profamily, proreligion, and protradition.

Gbadegesin, like Garcia, offers a careful philosophical analysis of the idea of culture and its moral implications in chapter 2. He is particularly concerned with the moral weight to be given cultural beliefs and practices, especially when they are in conflict. As evidence he compares and contrasts the narratives of three different African cultures, each with its particular values sometimes in significant conflict. He illustrates that Africa's cultures are themselves diverse and not monolithic.

Gbadegesin believes that all cultural practices should be accorded respect as a prima facie principle. However, he argues further that cultural beliefs cannot be self-justifying. When they come into conflict with each other, some ordering principle is required to resolve the conflict if decisions are to be made. Gbadegesin proposes this be a "principle of adjudication," which denies equal consideration to any cultural belief that impairs or impedes human flourishing. By "flourishing" he means the capacity to engage in community activity as a free person endowed with dignity.

In various ways the other essayists add specific content to Garcia's concept of an epistemological stance. Dula and King, in chapters 3 and 4, respectively, document the persisting disparities in the health and health care of African Americans. Despite efforts of public and philanthropic organizations, disparities in morbidity, mortality, health status, housing, and education persist at unacceptable levels. Both writers perceive this to be the result of continuing racism in America. Even though it exists in more subtle forms, some of it even unintentional, the idea of racism and all it connotes exerts continuing influence in African American life. Dula is very specific in describing the negative impact of the petrochemical, pharmaceutical, and tobacco industries on the health of black Americans.

In chapter 5, Sanders shows how racism and discrimination, as well as the memories of the Tuskegee and other unethical experiments, affected the response of African American postal workers to the anthrax threat. She links the extraordinary rate of refusal of proffered treatment to a deep distrust of health professionals and institutions. She also recognizes that African traditions, mores, and folkways also played a role especially in the preference for prayer and divine help, as well as folk remedies.

The epistemological stance is given personalized description in the autobiographical and reflective accounts by Griffith, a psychiatrist (chapter 6), and Peniston, a cardiac surgeon (chapter 7). Both are eminently successful in practice and academia. In his own way, each describes how the African American experience constructed a moral foundation for his own professional identity. Griffith emphasizes how the church, the challenge of authentically representing his own culture, and the dominant/nondominant tensions shaped his career. As a psychiatrist, Griffith is especially sensitive to the subtler nuances of being a member of the nondominant minority.

Peniston, conversely, points out that the African American perspective is not homogeneous. He contrasts the perspective and acceptance of Anglo-American values by some prominent African Americans—from extreme liberalism to extreme conservatism. Peniston calls for better scientific and empirical descriptions of what African Americans actually believe and practice. With these data he warns against simplistic group caricatures. In no way denying the realities of discrimination in his personal development, he calls for a more nuanced interpretation of the idea of the epistemological stance.

The concept of "race" is woven into the fabric of all of the essays. In chapter 8, FitzGerald and Royal look for the scientific foundations of that concept in modern biology, particularly in genetics. They believe, like Patricia King, that the concept may be useful rhetorically. However, they cannot find support for the concept of race anywhere in the vast amount of information now available about how humans are constituted biologically. The empirical and scientific existence of race and its putative relation with culture remains problematic.

Some Implications for Other Cultural Groups

The evidences of an African American perspective on bioethics provided in both volumes are specific and unique to the African American. There are, however, implications of a more general nature, relevant to the experiences of other cultural groups. The perspectives of Native Americans, for example, may perhaps be most closely related—particularly with respect to color discrimination, deprecation of human dignity, and possession of strong traditional folkways and medicine. Of a different order would be the current experiences of the many recent immigrant groups now entering America, legally and illegally, such as Latinos, Hispanics, Middle Easterners, and Asians. Each of these groups holds cultural beliefs that may conflict with the Anglo-American value set of contemporary bioethics. Most also have had adverse experiences of some kind with the dominant culture in their initial and continuing contacts with that culture.

The moral implications are not the same for African Americans and these other groups. They are similar enough, however, to generate analogous moral challenges for health professionals. These challenges are most concretely and urgently manifested in clinical decisions where decisions must be made and some resolution of conflict is mandatory.

Here the intersections between culture and ethics are often acute and complex. On one side are the beliefs and practices of the patient's cultural orientation. On the other are the ethics of the profession in question, the way the professional sees her professional moral obligations, and the culture of contemporary bioethics itself. In clinical encounters, the resolution of conflict is complicated by urgency and the emotional responses of both patient and professional.

Health professionals clearly have a moral obligation to respect the person of the patient no matter how far apart the cultural distance may be. Nonetheless, respect for persons does not entail an obligation on the part of the professional to violate her own professional or personal moral integrity. How to preserve both is becoming a source of anguish for caregivers.

Understanding the basis for distrust of health professionals and the health care system is essential. This means paying special attention to building trust, being faithful to promises, and removing any basis for a suspicion of discrimination. Special efforts to explain the nature of procedures, benefits and risks of treatments, and the identities and roles of members of the health care team are first steps. Additional attention must be given to making important decisions in the presence of distrust without peremptory resentment or taking of offense.

Individual practitioners cannot by themselves eradicate the persistent disparities of health care emphasized by the essayists. A reasonable modicum of pro bono work is a moral obligation of all health professionals. Collectively, however, health professionals have obligations through their professional associations to be advocates for removing injustices in availability, accessibility, and quality of services that African American and other groups might experience. If health professionals appreciated the moral power their collective advocacy could exert, they would feel less unable to effect change.

With respect to customs, beliefs, and practices with roots in African folkways related to illness and medicine, a more nuanced moral response is in order. The use of folk medicines and other treatments outside the perimeters of Western scientific or cosmopolitan medicine must be examined on an individual basis. Each must be evaluated from the point of harms they might produce for the patient. Some will be innocuous, some potentially dangerous, and some decidedly toxic. Likewise, some customs may be tolerable in certain circumstances, others not.

Cultural beliefs lie on a spectrum that extends from the benign to the totally indefensible. At the benign end are treatments that rely not on medication but on personal interactions, ritual, and so forth, whose content is known to be harmless. Some customs can, for good reason, be permitted at particular times, such as withholding information about lethal disease in cultures where this is customary and where the patient understands that this is what is happening. In some cases, the "therapeutic privilege" might be invoked. The same is true in cultures in which families or groups participate in decision making or actually make the decision instead of the patient. Consultation with native healers could fit this category if medication is not involved. Customs at the totally unacceptable end of the spectrum include ritual mutilation, gender selection by infanticide, abandonment of the elderly, ritual suicide or homicide, and so on. At this end of the spectrum, health professionals are expected to refuse any involvement, no matter how culturally entrenched the practice might be.

In the minds of many, religion is often associated with culture. As Sanders and Griffith attest in their essays, religion is an important element in the African American perspective. Whether religion is a separate category from other cultural practices is not a question to be settled here. It is clear, however, that in the cultural perspectives of most Americans, religion plays a significant role. Clearly, too, its moral weight as seen within most perspectives is of a higher order than other cultural elements. The foundations for religious moral norms are in theology, and their authority derives from a source beyond and above man. Religious belief thus has a special "weight" morally.

In the case of religion, the conflict is more apt to be between and among divergent religious beliefs than with academic and professional bioethics, which is pointedly secular and a-religious. This is a problem for all religions. So far as the obligations of health professionals go, there is an obligation to respect the dignity of each person but not necessarily his or her religious belief. This cannot mean submergence of the health professional's own beliefs. Rather, the professional must decide whether he or she can accommodate or compromise a patient's religious beliefs. If not, the professional should not enter the professional relationship, or should withdraw if the conflict is irresolvable. Under no circumstances, however, can the health professional use standards and norms of contemporary bioethics to impose alien beliefs or his or her own beliefs on the patient.

Two Fundamental Questions

The essays in this volume, and the discourse about the relations between bioethics and culture, raise two fundamental questions in moral philosophy that will occupy ethicists for some time to come. One is whether acceptance of the importance and reality of cultural diversity entails acceptance of moral relativism. The other is whether ethics and mores (culture, custom) are essentially different, and how.

Moral relativism comes in several forms.[10] For the sake of this discussion two types will suffice—strong moral relativism and weak relativism. Both begin with the indubitable empirical fact of moral diversity as an integral feature of cultural diversity, that is, different cultures hold different views about right and wrong, good and bad.

The strong version of moral relativism concludes from the empirical fact of diversity that there is no set of universal norms that can be validly applied to human life in any universal way. Each set of norms is valid only within the values and moral framework within which it resides and only within that framework. Further, there is no way to judge one set of moral beliefs against any others so that the idea of a universal set of principles is invalid. Discourse between and among cultural beliefs is impossible. The only recourse is respect for autonomy in secular ethics.[11]

The weak version of moral relativism also begins with the fact of cultural diversity. On this view there are obvious differences in religious practices and customs, but not necessarily in moral principles. Principles are the most fundamental sources for judgment of right and wrong, good and evil. This view distinguishes moral rules and practices from moral principles. The former may differ, but the latter do not, and thus principles form the basis for the judgment of a culture.[12] There may be differences between cultures on rules and practices and agreement on principles. The weak form of moral relativism allows for meaningful discourse among and between cultures as well as dialogue on the principles underlying the differences in rules and practices. The strong form precludes such a discussion.

Moral absolutism, on the other hand, holds that despite the enormous empirical diversity of moral beliefs, there are universal norms that apply to all humans. This is the classical ethical approach, and it is based in the acceptance of the idea of common human nature or essence. Moral discourse between and among divergent cultures consists in discovering and agreeing upon the universal norms common to the good life for all humans.

With the strong form of moral relativism, there is no way to judge the moral status of culture. Whatever a culture, society, group, or organization accepts as its customs and practices is what determines its morals. All cultures have equal weight. Without a universal criterion of moral judgment, culture itself is absolutized. Taken at full value, cultural absolutism is paradoxically the inevitable conclusion of moral relativism. Culture on this view is resistant to ethical analysis.

As to the second question about the relationship of a morality and ethics, there is a similar problem. If there is no basis for the judgment of a culture, then there is no discipline of ethics except within the narrow confines of each culture itself. Culture becomes self-justifying. Alternatively, if there is a difference between mores seen as habits with respect to right and wrong, then ethics becomes the instrument whereby the rightness and wrongness of culture can be examined. Ethics then can function as the discipline that critically, formally, and systematically studies morals, customs, and mores.

The relationships between ethics and morals are, of course, more complex than this.[13] The distinction offered here has proven helpful in resolving, or at least debating, the moral weight given to a given custom or practice. Gbadegesin suggests a principle of flourishing as the criterion. Michael Brannigan suggests a prima facie obligation to respect culture, allowing for culture to be trumped, although he is not specific about the criteria for trumping it. I would make the criterion the natural law, interpreted in the classical sense as that which defines what is common to man as man, that which makes man the kind of being he is.

None of these criteria for assessing the moral weight of custom or culture will be entirely convincing. Much more attention needs to be given to how ethics as a formal and critical discipline can survive when cultural diversity becomes more generally taken into account as it should be in making ethical decisions.

In this sense, ethics begins when culture becomes the subject of ethical analysis, that is, when its presuppositions are challenged. On this view, all customs and cultures would receive their justification by ethical examination. Bioethics intersects with culture at every turn, and this is where ethics and mores meet. If the fact of diversity is taken as justification for moral relativism in the strong sense, ethics is suborned by custom. If moral relativism of the weak type is accepted, then metacultural criticism is possible, and cultural diversity and moral norms are compatible.

Given the global nature of bioethics today, the profundity of the questions it must address and the multiplicity of cultures offering different perspectives in culture-free ethics can only end in moral chaos. To understand better how diversity relates to ethics, more empirical studies will help but will not answer the fundamental questions of moral philosophy. Lacking objective criteria for judgment, cultural diversity tends to become cultural hegemony often by violent means—as the world history has so often attested.

The critiques offered by the African Americans in this volume present serious moral challenges to bioethicists and health professionals. They are significant on their own account; they are also significant as an emerging crucial world problem—one with practical and theoretical implications for the ethical decisions of individuals and society.

The challenge of Harley Flack more than a decade ago in the first volume is even more urgent today: "Finding the keys to better multicultural relations is an imperative for global survival."[14]

Notes

1. Frederick M. Barnard, "Culture and Civilization in Modern Time," in *Dictionary of the History of Ideas*, vol. 1, ed. P. P. Weiner (New York: Charles Scribner's, 1973), 613–21.

2. A. L. Kroeber and Clyde Kluckhohn, *Culture* (New York: Meridian Books, 1952).

3. A. Kuper, *Culture: The Anthropologists' Account* (Cambridge, MA: Harvard University Press, 1999), 227.

4. Patricia Marshall and Barbara Koenig, "Accounting for Culture in Globalized Bioethics," *Journal of Law, Medicine and Ethics* 32 (2004): 252–66; Catherine Myser, "Differences from Somewhere: The Normativity of Whiteness in Bioethics in the United States," *American Journal of Bioethics* 3 (2003): 1–11; Charles Taylor, *Multiculturalism: Examining the Politics of Recognition* (Princeton, NJ: Princeton University Press, 1992).

5. Edmund Pellegrino, "Bioethics as an Interdisciplinary Enterprise: Where Does Ethics Fit in the Mosaic of Disciplines?" in *Philosophy of Medicine and Bioethics: A Twenty-Year Retrospective and Critical Appraisal*, ed. Ronald Carson and Chester R. Burns, *Philosophy and Medicine*, vol. 50 (Dordrecht: Kluwer, 1997), 1–24.

6. Daniel Callahan, "The Social Sciences and the Task of Bioethics," *Daedalus* 128 (1999): 275–94; Ruth Macklin, *Against Relativism: Cultural Diversity and Search for Ethical Universals in Medicine* (New York: Oxford University Press, 1999).

7. Harley E. Flack and Edmund D. Pellegrino, *African-American Perspectives on Biomedical Ethics* (Washington, DC: Georgetown University Press, 1992).
8. Edmund Pellegrino, P. Corsi, and Patricia Mazzarella, *Transcultural Dimensions in Medical Ethics* (Frederick, MD: University Publishing Group, 1992).
9. Joseph R. Betancourt, "Cultural Competence: Marginal or Mainstream Movement?" *New England Journal of Medicine* 351 (2004): 953–54.
10. Michael C. Brannigan, *Ethics across Cultures* (New York: McGraw-Hill, 2005), 13–28.
11. H. Tristram Engelhardt, *The Foundations of Bioethics*, 2nd ed. (New York: Oxford University Press, 1996).
12. Brannigan, *Ethics across Cultures*, 20.
13. William Frankena, *Ethics* (Englewood Cliffs, NJ: Prentice Hall, 1963); Bernard Williams, *Ethics and the Limits of Philosophy* (Cambridge, MA: Harvard University Press, 1985), 182–83.
14. Harley E. Flack, "The Confluence of Ethics and Culture," in *African-American Perspectives on Biomedical Ethics*, ed. Harley E. Flack and Edmund D. Pellegrino (Washington, DC: Georgetown University Press, 1992), xi.

CHAPTER 1

Revisiting African American Perspectives on Biomedical Ethics: Distinctiveness and Other Questions

Jorge L. A. Garcia

W H A T could make for a perspective on medical ethics that might be mean-ingfully and helpfully described as African American? Such a point of view might be distinguished by (a) its topics, for example, a focus on the distrib-ution of services and their delivery to the poor, or on certain illnesses dis-proportionately common or severe among African Americans (e.g., breast and prostate cancer, diabetes, sickle-cell anemia, hypertension); (b) its methodology, contrasting with a two-stage approach (first describing and then justifying "common morality," as advocated by Bernard Gert, Charles Culver, and K. D. Clouser[1]), for example, with a principlist method (in the man-ner of Tom Beauchamp and James Childress), with a casuistical/analogical pro-cedure (as found in Albert Jonsen and Stephen Toulmin), and a nonreduc-tionist form of role-professional ethics; (c) the principles, virtues, or values at work, as in Cheryl Sanders's claims about African American culture; or (d) some unique claims it makes about the morality (superiority, require-ment, wrongness, viciousness, etc.) of certain medical practices, and so on.

Certain difficulties, however, confront each of these. As to the first, (a), any theory or system of medical ethics ought to be comprehensive, with application to all relevant issues. Moreover, specialized focus seems to yield a medical ethical perspective on the health issues of an ethnoracial group, not an ethnoracial perspective on medical ethics. On (b), the claim that there is a distinctive methodology that is peculiar to African Americans is sociologically dubious, because it presupposes that there is something like a single culture shared by all and only African Americans—a difficult position to maintain in the face of manifest and growing intragroup diversity—and also dubious to the extent that it presupposes a now-discredited claim of racial essence.[2]

The same holds true for the claim, in (c), that there is a distinctive set of moral norms (rules, principles, values, virtues) specially embraced by (or otherwise proper to) African Americans.[3] Distinctive moral conclusions, on which (d) relies, would presumably have to be determined by application of a distinctive methodology, set of rules, and so forth, or by their application to a distinctive set of issues. So the viability of this option depends on that of one or more of the previous options.

Perhaps the most familiar way of interpreting an ethnoracial bioethical perspective depends on some form of cultural relativism, treating moral standards as inventions of cultures and as having application only within their founding culture's domain. However, a new set of problems about the understanding of culture has recently been raised against such cultural relativism.[4]

What is a culture or a cultural group? There is no single accepted account of the nature or identity conditions for a culture, and increasingly, specialists within social science and humanistic cultural studies see cultures as fluid, without clear boundaries, and internally variegated, even riven. (Edward Said has suggested we should abandon the commonplace that the human world is neatly divided into different social groups, each with its own distinctive culture.)[5]

In any case, there are other problems about cultures that must be overcome by the cultural relativist about morals. The "moral" norms supposedly internal to various cultures often seem to be (a) diversely distributed, with different people and subgroups espousing different claims; (b) sometimes indeterminate in content, lacking clear answers to some important questions; (c) contested within the cultural group; and (d) hierarchically imposed, with the powerful suppressing or silencing the voice of the powerless on what is right and wrong.[6]

These facts run contrary to relativists' frequent assumptions. They raise, first, problems of accuracy, for they indicate that there may often be no clear answer to the relativist's question of what the moral rules (or values, etc.) of some group (call them the Gs) require, prohibit, or permit. There is no definitive way to determine, nor is there a clear answer to the question of who is to say, who the Gs are, what their norms are, how those norms are properly interpreted, and so on. In addition, they raise political problems: to hold that the Gs' rules or values require, prohibit, or permit action of a certain type may be to acquiesce, even cooperate, in the subordination of a subgroup. Bernard Williams's unusually careful version of relativism holds that ethical discourse is chiefly couched in "thick" terms and that these have proper and meaningful application only *within* groups.[7] So it is not that a certain moral judgment that is true of or with respect to a cultural group, the *G1*s, for example, is *false* for a different cultural group, the *G2*s, for example, as we are inclined to think a meaningful relativism must entail, but rather that this moral judgment has no application (and so is *not true*) for the *G2*s. Still, Williams's suggestion doesn't suffice to vindicate cultural relativism about morals. Many "thick" moral descriptions will have cross-cultural application. Of course, proscriptions against stealing or marital infidelity get no purchase in a society lacking private property or marriage. Still, even when they do not, we can ask why the preconditions are missing. Maybe their absence points to some moral failing (or advantage) in the society. In any case, the relevant norms could still be formulated as conditionals ("If people here come to have property or spouses, then it would be wrong . . ."), having meaningful application contingent on certain possibilities.[8]

What is important is not so much a medical ethics that is distinctive of African Americans as one that is faithful, informed by, and seriously responsive to important forms of experience characteristic of African Americans, that is, informed and responsive in its topics (foci), methods, moral features, or content.[9] Recent "standpoint epistemology," in its moderate forms, allows that a person's (or group's) vantage point may afford her (or them) an epistemic advantage in seeing things others miss.[10] Similarly, recent work in so-called virtue ethics allows that people sensitized in certain ways, by a regimen of cultivation but also by their experiences, may perceive morally significant features of a situation to which features others are blind.[11]

Looking Back

In a 1992 article on this topic, I offered several elements of a meaningfully African American medical ethics perspective. These included the claims that it should be (a) antimajoritarian and antiutilitarian, (b) antisituationist, and (c) distrustful of an "ethics of trust"; that it (d) regard the patient as the one with the decision to make; that it be (e) sympathetic toward families without romanticizing them; and that it remain (f) free from the bonds of scientism and (g) open to insights from religious faith. Related to this last point, and finally, I indicated that it (h) need not be beholden to the neutralist political liberalism that dominated elite political thought in the last century's final decades, which often revealed a strongly antireligious streak.

So conceived, everyone can and should learn from medical ethical reflection that is duly informed by consideration of experiences widespread among African Americans. Indeed, the chief importance of such an ethical perspective—that is, an approach duly informed by reflection on African American lives—is not as something self-sufficient but rather lies in what it can contribute to an overall view that takes cognizance of, and remains faithful to, a variety of such points of view. This and other particular perspectives matter chiefly as vantage points that yield vital input, but are ultimately to be transcended by their incorporation into a comprehensive moral vision.

Today, these claims still seem largely correct to me, though I wish now to state more clearly that these elements are ones I think *ought* to characterize an approach to medical ethics that learns (some of) the *right* lessons from African American experiences. I do not mean to advance a value-free description. I will attempt no detailed interpretation of African American history, lives, and experiences, nor offer any careful defense of my view that it justifies the features of bioethical reflection I have claimed can be grounded in it (as well as grounded in other ways). Rather, I will indicate aspects of that history in support of each such feature.

Such a stance would, in summary, center on the essential and inviolable dignity of the human person. From there and for that reason, it should, contrary to majoritarianism and consequentialism, refuse to sacrifice one for the sake of others, insisting no less on the solidarity whereby all place themselves in jeopardy for the sake of any one. It should view and assess any human action, individual or collective, by the citizen or the state, on the basis of the sort of response that action manifests to that unique status, not on the basis of the action's mere effects—actual, probable, or expected. It hardly needs to be said why people who have been subjugated as an ethnic minority for the benefit of others should see through, even if some ethical theorists cannot, any claim that benefit to the "greatest number" suffices to justify action. Similarly, it should be particularly plain to people whose victimization has sometimes been defended as a form of compassionate paternalism that any goodwill from which others act needs always to be combined with respectful deference and appreciation of their essential human status and dignity.[12]

Against situationism and cultural relativism, this stance needs to insist that any chosen course be rationally defensible, not merely presented as a given required, in some inarticulable way, by the demands of the situation and which we are to accept on trust in the educated and professional classes. We, whose great-grandfathers were enslaved in accordance with state law, ought to have learned that local norms provide little guarantee of equitable treatment and that a greater measure of protection is accorded when actions have to be justified publicly and in accordance with widely recognized universal moral principles.

Likewise, calls to trust the educated and professional have to be seen as aspirational until that trust is earned. It may be, as some moral theorists rightly maintain, that the agent's virtue is a surer indicator of moral action than are any rules. Still, the problem is that we should know better than to think that social privilege reliably predicts personal virtue.

Individualism certainly has its flaws and is often taken to an unjustifiable extreme in American legal, political, and moral thinking. Nevertheless, contrary to the rhetoric of radical anti-individualism, communitarianism, and identitarianism, we African Americans—who have often become invisible to others, disappearing beneath a perceived black mask—should know that it is in persons alone that human dignity resides and that their human identity always transcends any such parochial association. Indeed, the various forms and levels of community (not just racial, but also national and religious, generational and epochal) are important for what they contribute to the lives of particular persons. Moreover, while rightly spurning dangerously unrealistic views of the family, people with histories like ours ought to recognize the life of any human person as necessarily involved with those of others. We should not have to be tutored into appreciating family, neighborhoods, self-help organizations, political alliances, and the other ties that constitute the mediating institutions of civil society. Because the black church has been such a source of solidarity and political activism, as well as a source of moral insight for members of the white majority, those taking such a stance should know enough to repudiate the hostility toward religion so common among leftist intellectuals. African Americans may be unusually well situated to recognize that any such moral stance on the stature and importance of human beings can draw inspiration, formation, and support from a rightly conceived understanding of the human person in her nature and vocation. That opens such an ethical perspective to due influence and shaping by religious reflection.

Because the late twentieth-century's neutralist liberalism, overly impressed by the less and less relevant story of early modern Europe's intra-Christian wars, is a prime locus of such antireligious hostility, it should also give this approach moral purchase to resist the blandishments of that liberalism's illegitimate demand for an impossible and indefensible state neutrality across conceptions of how to live and, still worse, its attempts to silence religious voices in the public arena. Reflecting on the differing but interrelated stories of Africans in America should make us tremble to think how much longer slavery and Jim Crow would have survived but for the moral outcry and social action by those—both leaders and followers, black and white—driven by their religious convictions to voice their moral insight in the public forum.

Looking Forward

I venture to suggest that several parts of today's thought stand much to gain from a bioethical perspective properly informed in the ways just sketched. First, African American political discussion could benefit from an intellectual stance infused with these elements from a reflection on the lessons of African American experiences. Too often, our black political thought still confines itself to the imaginary beings and fanciful determinants of Marxist social theory, or descends into the destructive and divisive illusions of the politics of identity and authenticity.[13] A bioethical perspective and more general approach to normative matters that is informed in the ways I have indicated would enable us more firmly to contextualize political activism and root it realistically in needed moral considerations. Interestingly, some European and "Euro-American" thinkers of the radical left have recently returned to ancient and even medieval moral reflection on human nature, destiny, flourishing, and virtue as a way to rethink politics in the aftermath of Soviet Communism's political demise and Marxism's increasing moral and intellectual discredit.[14] Perhaps incorporating elements from such a way of thinking about bioethics into broader thinking about ethical and political matters would broaden discussion among black intellectuals, freeing it from the constraints of late nineteenth- and twentieth-century socioeconomic pieties and predictable ideological placement.

Second, today's bioethical thinking can also benefit from such a humanizing influence. Too often the regnant schools of thought within the field, whatever their internecine differences over methodological arcana, merely serve as local outposts of late modernist liberalism. That is, they seldom transcend concern with vague abstractions about "quality of life" and an instrumentalizing consequentialist caricature of moral deliberation, cloaked in the pseudorational rhetoric of values "balancing." They are prone to deny the essential healing nature of medicine or to twist it into fitting within a single-minded mania for relieving discomfort, even as a rationalization for medical homicide. Moreover, they are given to conceptions of autonomy divorced from Kant's insistence on freeing the self from its passions and subjecting it to the internal discipline of reason and tend toward a radical secularism that sometimes becomes antireligious.[15] Increasingly, commercial interest is allying itself with ideology to narrow the range of opinion, as bioethicists work for corporations, nonprofits, trade associations, and other institutions that want only regulatory niceties but have little use for ethical condemnation of important parts of their business. (Consider the problematic employment of staff bioethicists by, among others, health maintenance organizations [HMOs], for-profit and not-for-profit hospitals, the biotechnology industry, and "reproductive health" or genetics counseling operations and their associations.) Indeed, even ethics researchers affiliated with university-based or independent research centers in ethics or biomedicine may feel economic pressure to tailor their opinions, as their institutions rely on and compete to please corporations (and corporate-founded or -funded philanthropic foundations) for what are demurely designated "gifts" to endow chairs, fund programs, establish and maintain laboratories, and so on.

For such reasons, the "ethicist" often functions chiefly to confer the *imprimatur* of rationality and morality on decisions driven by cost-consciousness, on degrading biotechnological innovations rooted in some scientists' hubris, and on a variety of subjective whims, quirks, and kinks they wrongly exalt as exercises of an autonomy that would be unrecognizable to Kant, the concept's chief expositor, as well as on other elements of an unworthy social agenda.[16] I fear it will take some future satirist—a new Aristophanes or Swift to arise in the decades ahead—to capture adequately the grotesque effrontery of our time, when it is precisely in the universities' self-proclaimed centers of ethics and values that credentialed "ethicists" opine that some human beings are nonpersons, without rights or even lives worth our saving (or restraining ourselves from taking), and actively promote ever-new programs of homicide against the most deprived and vulnerable, those with least power.

Third, this thinking could help align some black ethical bioethical thought with, and therein support, some of the important criticisms raised by voices from the disability rights movement who reject the application of (and sometimes the theory behind) quality of life (QOL) assessment and other commonplaces within today's degraded, antilife bioethics. This would be admirably countercultural in speaking love, dignity, and truth to the hegemony of complacent and powerful academic and institutional orthodoxies.

Finally, today's medical research and practice should also likely benefit from being informed by a bioethical perspective such as the one I have suggested African American experiences properly support.[17] With concierge medicine, rule by so-called HMOs, and similar abuses now growing, a return to core insights about the nature of medicine and responsible moral reasoning can only help.[18]

The Use of Racial Concepts in Medical Research

The legitimacy of using racial categories in medical research is controversial today, chiefly because of larger misgivings about the legitimacy—linguistic and conceptual, social and political—of racial classification.[19] Today's philosophical theorists have raised numerous doubts about the viability of the concept of race. Thus Anthony Appiah holds that the findings of current genetic biology vindicate neither "ideational" nor "referential" understandings of the language of race.[20] Naomi Zack believes that the same holds true of cultural anthropology, population genetics, philosophy of science, and other related inquiries.[21] Joshua Glasgow holds that "cladistic" biological accounts, which stress reproductive groups and practices in contrast to genetic/molecular approaches, fail to restore a scientifically respectable account of race.[22]

For all that, some philosophers have devised partial defenses of race. Thus Lucius Outlaw thinks racial thinking may play a natural part in reproductive decisions.[23] That is the reason, he believes, that those with access to intercontinental travel are not all tan-colored by now. His position is not unproblematic. The appeal he makes fails to show that race itself is real, only that racial thinking is deep rooted. Philip Kitcher advances a view somewhat like Outlaw's, holding that race may be both socially and biologically real, because it impacts reproductive behavior.[24] Again, there is a problem, for he simply presupposes, without offering or defending, answers to the hard questions of racial classification.

Perhaps Michael Hardimon gives a way out for the devotee of race. He thinks that the core "concept" of race (as reproductively transmitted gross morphological features originating and varying with Continental land masses) can be separated from familiar but dubious "conceptions," in such a way as to license the former's retention.[25] Still, it is controversial whether biology licenses even this minimal core of race. David Wasserman's case amounts to what logicians call a *tu quoque* argument. Wasserman suggests that while race is conceptually problematic, so are species. If we legitimately retain the latter within biological science, so too may race be justified.[26] Still, this does not settle the issue. Even if Wasserman is correct that scientific recourse to the category of species is more problematic than is usually acknowledged, the cases are not on a par for ethics. Without some classification such as that of species there can be no sense given to claims that an organism is better or worse off. For whether equipping an animal with wings or fins, for example, is a benefit to it, improves its life, or helps it to function depends on whether it is bird or a fish. Thus neither consequentialist nor nonconsequentialist moral theories would have application. No case can be made that race is similarly necessary for ethical reasoning. To mention just one additional position, Paul Taylor offers a self-consciously pragmatist approach to these questions. He maintains that dropping race talk would mask commonalities among, and the etiology of, much social deprivation.[27] One trouble with this argument is that showing we need to remember that the serious social impact on people of being widely classified and treated as members of the black race does not guarantee that this or any other race is real. It is just an abuse of the legitimate but very limited notion of social construction (or, better, social constitution) to hold that someone's being widely judged an S means that she is an S or even that any Ss exist. We should be familiar with enough erroneous classifications and illusory categories to avoid that trap.

In the end, it remains uncertain whether we can safely repudiate race as scientifically bogus. The chief line of response from those who defend the existence of races and our continued employment of racial classification differs from the quasi-biological or metaphysical positions we have just noted. They reconceive race as "socially real," not "biologically real," as some put the point. We cannot adequately explore this option here, but I wish to register some overlooked obstacles to the increasingly common move of regarding race as a "social construction."

First, if it is socially constructed, then a person's race would vary when she moved from one society to another with a relevantly different scheme of racial categorization, and even when she was differently thought of in her own society. This is quite different from how we ordinarily employ the concept. Even if we allow that someone's race could change, we seem to require a deep change in her, in her body, not simply in the minds of other people. Second, social construction presupposes and requires the preexistence of persons, social groups, social procedures, and so on. It cannot go "all the way down," contrary to the extreme views of such thinkers as Richard Rorty, for then there would be no constructors to begin the process of construction. Yet race, if it exists at all, would seem to be something built into a person, not a status she comes to have. Third, social construction makes little sense when not restricted to categories or roles that are intrainstitutional, qualitative (not entitative), and limited to having various rights and privileges. Your being a judge or a student can be socially constituted because it consists in your having a certain role within our institutional practices, and it is plainly up to us to assign rights and duties within those. However, races are not similarly institutional or exclusively normative features, even if some people have normative expectations of those assigned to various races.

A second way of defending our retention and continued reliance on racial categories, one not entirely distinct from appeal to social construction, is to *replace* race with racial identity. Without attempting to examine this option fully, we should at least note several difficulties in viewing race as a group/social identity. Some are conceptual difficulties. Socially constructed race would vary too much and be too external to the self to count meaningfully as identity. For anyone's identity should comprise only what is (a) essential to the person, (b) limited to fields (e.g., being identical in color), (c) relational (or relationally formulable: "This is identical to that"), (d) perdurant through change ("It is *this* that perdured while one height, age, and so on passed way and it came to be characterized by another"), and (e) conceptually tied to sameness. It is striking and problematic that not one of these holds true of supposed racial or ethnic identities.

Other difficulties for this sort of identity theory are political, moral, or social. Racial identity as a personal quest or group project—that is, as a quest for a supposed authenticity—is troubling because it can tend to rely on stereotypes, which are factually dubious; privilege some subgroups over others; often be socially dangerous; presuppose a doubtful authenticity; stifle individuality; suppress creativity, often to the group's (as well as the individual's) detriment; and breed political division.[28]

Of course, none of this is to deny that socially *caused* differences among people can matter, whether or not there are biological or socially *constructed* (i.e., socially constituted) races. Causation is very different from constitution. Industrial pollution, for example, is caused by us, through our socially licensed or ignored practices and policies, and it causes us to be sick. Yet neither pollution nor disease is a social construction, because neither consists in people's sharing or coordinating their beliefs, resolutions, or agreements. Still, that causation may be all that is needed for some limited reliance upon racial categories in medical research.

The concept of race is, at best, intellectually problematic, and we well know that it has been implicated in horrifying forms of sociopolitical degradation and victimization. Must we, then, reject its employment in, for example, the recent suggestion that certain drugs, which have manifested differential effectiveness across racial groups, be recommended and prescribed for patients in some racial groups but not others? That conclusion is, I think, both hasty and too strong. Rather, it seems to me that two recent scientific commentators have offered the right sort of response. David Goldstein and Huntington Willard, in an op-ed piece, sensibly submit that "the FDA may well be justified in approving BiDil [one such drug] for use in African-Americans," because research indicated in the 1980s that it worked rather well on African Americans but with otherwise unimpressive results.[29] However, they note that this will pose the practical problem for the physician of determining just who is and who is not African American and caution that any such "use of race in clinical medicine is an interim, and frankly unfortunate, measure that society should replace." They urge that research continue "to clarify the [nonracial] factors that underlie the drug's selective effectiveness," factors that may well have more to do with the different chemical environments to which those differently classified by race are exposed, and describe race ("skin color") as "imperfect indicators."[30] While I am somewhat less confident that racial classification will ultimately prove unsustainable, I agree with these two genome scientists that such reliance on racial categories in medical science ought for now to be temporary, provisional, reluctant, non-committal, admitted as crude, and occurring only in concert with continued research to identify more precisely the real causal factors at work.

Some Ethnoracial Issues in Medical Ethics: Queries and Suggested Directions

Let us turn now from this to some other ethical issues in medical inquiry, practice, and institutions. We should look to how an improved bioethical perspective might help illuminate some current controversies. I will briefly raise three and pose some questions and indicate paths for exploration: transracial disparities[31] in health and health care, the problem of black mistrust of the medical profession, and the challenge of new reproductive (and antireproductive) technologies.

First, then, racial disparity in levels of health, susceptibility to various illnesses, health care access, medical prescription and treatment, and elsewhere are now well documented and widely discussed.[32] The primary ethical question is "What type of moral objection is properly raised against the practices that help produce these racial disparities, and wherein does it lie?"[33] Our intuitive response is likely to be that these disparities strike us as unjust. If so, why? Perhaps simply because they are unequal. But then it needs to be clarified whether the needed equality is one that holds across *persons* or, what is quite different, across *races*. (Even if some individuals have a claim-right to receive better care or a liberty-right to acquire it, that is not the same as a moral requirement that there be no disparities across races.) Again, we need ethical clarification on whether it is the *existence* of this inequality that is objectionable morally, or its *magnitude*. Is the inequality unjust simply as a characteristic of a slice of time, or is it the historical context of past oppression of African Americans that is morally crucial?

Perhaps the disparities are unjust because they are *unfair* rather than because they are simply unequal. Is what matters, then, that they do or do not result from some bias or cheating or exploitation in the relevant procedures? Or is it instead that they are unfair because they deprive African Americans of what we are owed as a matter of compensatory justice? Maybe the moral problem is that some people are—or that the racial group as a whole is— left below some minimum morally acceptable standard of welfare.[34]

But perhaps the disparities matter morally not so much as violations of individual rights but because of what they mean for social comity. If so, is it their deleterious *effects* on the prospects for future comity or fraternity that make the disparities morally unacceptable? Or is it that they are signs and products of a historical or current absence of sentiments and acts of social solidarity? Or is it that, whatever in fact happens to result, any line of reasoning that serves to justify these disparities would also justify other social arrangements even more clearly divisive and inimical to an important sense of shared mission?

My own suggestion is that the issue of injustice cannot be answered by simply observing and recording statistical disparities. Rather, we need to see how they arise and are maintained—more specifically, what matters for justice is whether they stem from the disrespect that lies at the heart of social or personal injustice. There are, after all, no unjust situations as such, only unjust choices and the unjust actions that arise from them. Conversely, even if the disparities' origin or continuance do not issue from such disrespect, and are therefore not unjust, they may nonetheless be socially problematic because they violate the sense of shared mission and shared fate any stable society needs if it is to constitute and maintain itself as a community.

Second, there are problems arising from the mistrust of medical professionals and their institutions. Some thinkers have attributed part of the health disparity to African Americans' being less inclined to follow their doctors' orders. Others have pushed further and attributed such reluctance, if it exists, to a broader distrust of medical professionals and institutions, which has been indicated in other studies.

Who properly bears the burden of rectifying this distrust? Is it up to African Americans ourselves to develop habits and attitudes that are likely to prove beneficial in the long run? Should the health care establishments acknowledge a responsibility to build trust, especially in light of events such as the infamous Tuskegee syphilis study, which have helped destroy it?[35] Is this distrust irrational, or does the history provide significant warrant for it and show that there are serious risks, as well as benefits, in African Americans' placing greater trust in health care professionals?[36]

Again, I will not attempt here to resolve these controversies. However, I can say that it seems to me that the medical profession—in its members, practices, organizations, and institutions—needs to acknowledge its substantial share of the blame for widespread black mistrust in this country and take serious steps to redress it, reaching out to underserved groups entitled to, but ambivalent about, greater care, treatment, and instruction about health.

Third, consider some of the new reproductive technologies currently envisioned or already becoming possible. I have in mind nightmarish scenarios—where people are designed according to our specifications to be able to concentrate beyond distraction, perform more efficiently, never grow old, stay thin and fit, maintain youthful skin and eyesight, forget only what they choose to, and remain cheerful through it all—that pose serious questions.[37] Does the endeavor to realize these visions amount to treating people as mere means to chosen ends, reminiscent of the worst abuses in twentieth century medical research? And what of the various means to their realization? Are some humans being destroyed and dismembered for experimentation because of their physical differences (their overall size and shape this time, rather than their skin color and the shape of particular features) and their level of capacity? If so, have Americans adequately learned the lessons of our history of black slavery and racial discrimination? What messages to and about African Americans are implicit in the human ideals underlying these designs? What will be the social effects of the likely unequal and racially disparate access to and possession of the new bioenhancements? How will feelings of shared fate and commonality across racial and other boundaries be affected once significant numbers of people have been bioengineered for enhancement and perform at the intended levels? What becomes of fair competition in the workplace, the schoolroom, the playing field, and elsewhere, once the ordinary and natural contest for advancement against the genetically enhanced?

I think an approach to medical ethics of the sort I have sketched here and elsewhere—a perspective informed by, among other things, reflection on and appropriation of important experiences of African people in America—should shake up today's underexamined ideological alliances and associations, in which those most concerned to end antiblack racism and reverse its effects, when they turn to medical ethics, tend to abandon their commitments to universal respect for humanity, the protection of every human being's rights and life, the dignity of each as prior to the interests of all or most, and a vision of our brotherhood and sisterhood as rooted in the Creator's fatherhood. In short, I think the quest to protect the defenseless at the beginning and end of human life from medical homicide—from euthanasia, suicide-enablement, infanticide, abortion, and embryo-destroying experiments—should be recognized as a logical and proper extension of our continuing struggles against racial violence and injustice. Of course, that requires us to get beyond the shallow journalistic polarities of left, right, conservatives, liberals, and radicals.

Conclusion

In this chapter I have sought, first, to clarify what I take to be an especially promising, illuminating, and helpful interpretation of the idea of African American perspectives on biomedical ethics. I have tried to indicate some of its promise for correcting several parts of our thought and practice and to come to terms with some objections raised against my earlier effort. I have also sketched and tried to apply lessons gleaned from a long-overdue philosophically sophisticated discussion of race, which has arisen since the 1992 volume on African American perspectives on biomedical ethics. Finally, descending a bit from theory toward practice, I have posed central questions for a medical ethics that confronts racial division and injustice and have indicated ways in which we should begin to answer them from a perspective properly informed by reflection on aspects of African people's experience in America. I hope to have challenged some familiar assumptions and political orthodoxies, sacred cows of many intellectuals, and to have provoked sometimes uncomfortable lines of thought. If I have succeeded in that, I will be satisfied that I have indicated some of the promise of exploring these perspectives and of both accommodating them and incorporating them within the viewpoints of medical ethics.

Notes

I am grateful to Dr. Prograis and the Georgetown University Center for Clinical Medical Ethics for inviting my contribution, and to an audience at a September 2004 Georgetown conference for questions and suggestions. My research was greatly facilitated by my 2003–5 appointments as a Nonresident Fellow in Harvard University's Du Bois Institute.

1. Bernard Gert, Charles Culver, and K. D. Clouser, *Bioethics: A Return to Fundamentals* (Oxford: Oxford University Press, 1997).
2. K. Anthony Appiah, "Race, Culture, and Identity: Misunderstood Connections," in *Color Conscious*, ed. K. Anthony Appiah and Amy Gutmann (Princeton, NJ: Princeton University Press, 1996), 30–105.
3. For a different view, see Sanders's contribution to this volume.

4. See Gbadegesin's contribution to this volume for a helpful and instructive historical discussion of changing conceptions of culture in the modernist epoch.

5. Adam Kuper, *Culture: The Anthropologists' Account* (Cambridge, MA: Harvard University Press, 1999), 221.

6. See, e.g., discussions in Kuper, *Culture*; Michele Moody-Adams, *Fieldwork in Familiar Places* (Cambridge, MA: Harvard University Press, 1997).

7. For Williams, these "thick" terms have substantial descriptive content that cannot neatly be prized away from their evaluative status.

8. See Putnam's critique of Williams for further discussion: Hilary Putnam, *Collapse of the Fact-Value Dichotomy* (Cambridge, MA: Harvard University Press, 2002).

9. Peter Singer's notorious analogy between racism and something he calls "speciesism" seems to me not a serious engagement but a simpleminded exploitation: Peter Singer, *Practical Ethics*, 2nd ed. (New York: Cambridge University Press, 1993). The suggestion that the difference between African and European peoples is anything like that between humans and lower animals is grotesque and offensive. In a combination of doubtful consistency, Richard Dawkins fulminates against "speciesism" while professing a zealot's devotion to evolutionary psychology. See Richard Dawkins, *A Devil's Chaplain* (Boston: Houghton Mifflin, 2003), and the thoughtful critique in Stephen Barr, "The Devil's Chaplain Confounded," *First Things* (August/September 2004): 25–30. I offer a critical overview of several aspects of Singer's thought and what its prominence says about the squalid state of much contemporary bioethics, in J. Garcia, "The Professor of Death: Peter Singer," *Books & Culture* (September/October 2001): 30–33.

10. Linda M. Alcoff, "Who's Afraid of Identity Politics?" in *Reclaiming Identity*, ed. Paula Moya and Michael Hames-Garcia (Berkeley: University of California Press, 2000), 312–44.

11. See Lawrence Blum, *Moral Perception and Particularity* (New York: Cambridge University Press, 1994).

12. I think that following this emphasis on the motivational input to action—respect, deference, appreciation, response—rather than its output (consequences), should help lead the ethical theorist out of the thickets of consequentialism into an understanding of moral life closer to what is called virtue ethics. However, that would take our inquiry far afield, and I will not pursue this point here.

13. I have in mind the elaborate Marxist mythology of capitalism's two necessary and constitutive classes, their supposedly inevitable clash to be resolved only in the romance of revolution, society's purported "ideological superstructure" resting on its economic base, the alleged exploitation of wage laborers by extracting "surplus value" from their work, and so forth. Some of Jon Elster's work

marks a helpful start on the overdue work of collapsing this intellectual house of cards: Jon Elster, *Making Sense of Marx* (New York: Cambridge University Press, 1985).

14. See Terry Eagleton, *After Theory* (New York: Basic Books, 2003). Also, Paul Griffiths, "Christ and Critical Theory," *First Things* (August/September 2004): 46–55, offers an interesting overview of other moves by nonbelievers on the socialist left to remake their politics by drawing on theological ethics and philosophical anthropology derived from classical Greek and medieval Christian sources. (He treats works of the last two decades by Jean-François Lyotard, Alain Badiou, and Slovaj Žižek, whose recent theorizing turns to Aristotle, the Gospels, Paul's epistles, Augustine, and Aquinas, among others.) It is ironic that though African Americans are among the most religious and politically vocal ethnic grouping in the United States, boasting some of the country's most prominent public intellectuals, comparatively little such movement toward regrounding radical left politics in religious and moral sources is evident. (Some of the work of Cornel West, a Protestant minister who blends Marxism and democratic socialist activism with Christian practice and preaching, is the most important theorizing of such synthesis among African American writers. For an introduction, see Cornel West, *The Cornel West Reader* [New York: Basic Books, 1999], esp. sections V, "Radical Democratic Politics," and VI, "Prophetic Christian Theology.") One danger, of course, is that such synthesis may fail to rise above incoherent syncretism or mere eclecticism. If such syntheses are unstable and a choice must finally be made, as I suspect, it is not clear to me why Far Left politics ought to command greater allegiance among those seeking to learn ethical lessons from African American life than do understandings of moral life, Christian and philosophical, focused on the virtues of character.

15. The President's Council on Bioethics, under the leadership of Drs. Leon Kass and Edmund Pellegrino, has been an important exception to these generalizations, and its reports and inquiries have helped point a different direction for medical ethics. Unfortunately, such is the politicization of the field that it is hard to be optimistic that many within it will follow that guidance and effectively reform the field.

16. For an analysis of the content and causes of the moral and intellectual deterioration of medical ethics over the twentieth century's last three decades, see J. Garcia, "Reforming Healthcare Ethics," in *Medical Ethics at Notre Dame*, ed. Margaret Hogan and David Solomon (Notre Dame, IN: University of Notre Dame Press, forthcoming). Also see Marcell Bombardieri and Gareth Cook, "Scientist: Racism Hurt Him at MIT," *Boston Globe,* January 14, 2005, pp. B1, B7, for discussion of a recent case that interestingly defies the usual expectations. They treat the charge of Dr. James Sherley that he was victimized by individual and institutionalized racism at MIT. While I venture no opinion on the merits

of Dr. Sherley's charge, what makes the case instructive is that he, a man described as son of a Baptist minister, opposes on moral grounds destructive experiments on humans who are at the embryonic stage. In preference to these horrors, committed to extract stem cells in hopes of advancing biological knowledge and eventually developing medical treatments, Dr. Sherley advances fuller inquiry into the use of adult stem cells, which can be harvested without taking the lives of embryonic humans. This decency predictably outrages some of his scientific peers, who can brook no ethical qualms about, objections to, or delay of their research agendas. To the extent that we have come to expect charges of antiblack racism to come from the political left, and moral criticism of embryo research to come from the Right, Dr. Sherley's case is useful in aiding us to think beyond these stereotypes. However, I think we should not be surprised if it turns out that those with no respect for human life at its most defenseless and vulnerable stages should also treat some adults with similarly disrespectful discrimination. Indeed, nothing should be less surprising.

17. Arthur Kleinman, "Anthropology of Bioethics," in *Writing at the Margin* (Berkeley: University of California Press, 1995), 88–89, and passim.

18. Revisiting these topics fifteen years later, I should address some criticisms that my 1992 views elicited. First, I treat the physician and anthropologist Arthur Kleinman's relativist critique of my antirelativism. It will be charged here that I tacitly rely on a nineteenth-century moralized conception of human culture. However, the recent dismantling of the variously murky twentieth-century conceptions requires some retrieval of clearer, more defensible understandings of culture if the notion of culture is not to be jettisoned altogether. On the concept's late twentieth-century's woes, see Kuper, *Culture*. Kleinman faults me for relying "on an idea of culture as beliefs, values, and judgments: conventions that can be taken up or put down at will." Regarding as "suspect" the "use of abstract concepts of justice and beneficence as universal ethical principles," he advocates "a constrained and engaged relativism," which recognizes "the cultural roots of ethical systems" but views cultures as themselves in flux.

In response to Kleinman, I first affirm that no serious person thinks that anyone's "beliefs, values, and judgments" are adopted or rejected "at will," of course, and nothing I have said commits me to such a preposterous claim. Nor is the issue whether cultures change over time, but whether what some take to be the group's norms are really there and are really theirs. Are they fully determinate in their content? Are they sufficiently clear in their interpretation and application? Do they belong to the whole group or only to some? Are they really endorsed by the group rather than controverted within it? Even if they are endorsed by the group, to what extent does this surface unanimity reflect inner conviction and not the illegitimate exercise of power in suppressing dissent? Even within Kleinman's "constrained" relativism, as I understand it, problems remain both in justifying the classification of these disputes as moral and in making sense of their content. Are they not arguing, after all, what they ought to permit, require, prohibit, and so on? But then that cannot be a dispute over what they already do permit, require, prohibit, and so on. In denying that "moral deliberations . . . transcend or avoid culture," Kleinman makes it clear that he regards moral reasoning as constituted and operating by varying cultural procedural patterns or rules. But because nothing can properly count as a human culture unless it cultivates and fulfills people, which is an ineluctably evaluative matter of fact, tying all standards to culture can only be circular.

Second, I take up Beauchamp's critique of my views of relativism, morality, and racial perspective. Tom Beauchamp, "Response to Jorge Garcia," in *African-American Perspectives on Biomedical Ethics*, ed. Harley E. Flack and Edmund D. Pellegrino (Washington, DC: Georgetown University Press, 1992), 67–73. Beauchamp makes three charges: (a) My antirelativism permits an unsatisfying "relativism of judgments" even if it rejects "relativism of standards"; (b) my antirelativist argument presupposes that "morality" is univocal, where he thinks it may instead be what philosophers call a "cluster concept," or "family resemblance" term, which corresponds to no one essence and is used with "many senses or at least . . . many diverse marks or criteria"; and (c) my account allows that the elements of an African American perspective are only "contingently and historically" tied to a particular ethnic group, in that other groups might have them (or have had them) and this group might not have.

Here are some responses to Beauchamp's criticisms. Expressing his doubts about my "relativity thesis," Beauchamp defines "cultural relativism [as] diversity of belief deriving from cultural diversity" and "[moral] judgments [as] acts of evaluating in which moral values or principles are clarified, specified, applied, or interpreted." So, *cultural* relativism of *moral* judgments, which seems to be what Beauchamp imputes to me, would be the claim that people sometimes make different moral judgments because they are influenced by their different cultures. That seems to me to affirm only cross-cultural diversity of moral opinion. I will not go into whether it is correct, though few would deny it. What matters is that it does not amount to cultural relativism about morality, not in any important sense. As I said in my 1992 article, serious cultural relativism about morals requires not just such belief in culturally induced *diversity* but also acceptance both of genuine *relativity* (so that moral judgments make sense or have validity only within, or with respect to, a certain culture) and of *nonhierarchy* (according to which the different moral views common in different cultures cannot be ranked as [more nearly] true or false).

Turning now to Beauchamp's misgivings about my view on the "concept of morality," I should clarify that my argument against relativism had two main claims. First, the advocate of strong moral relativism needs contrasting judgments to be so *similar* in content, bases, and so on that they can be properly classed as "moral" but also so *different* in content, bases, and so on that they can plausibly be said to represent incompatible moralities. Second, this combination is difficult to hold because it is unstable and in internal tension. Nothing in that position, contra Beauchamp, requires a strong and narrow essentialism about morality. All it demands is going beyond the shallow and lazy inference that if one group frequently engages in a practice and praises people for it, while another shuns and condemns the practice, then the difference between them must be a moral disagreement and a deep one. The divergence in practice is, of course, irrelevant, as it is not surprising or uncommon for people to do what they or other members of their society think immoral. This is true even if the first group only praises and never condemns the practice, and the other only condemns and never praises it, which goes beyond our initial stated hypothesis. Even in this latter case, the relativist would still need to show that the disagreement is about what is morally right and wrong. I doubt that Beauchamp, no fan of moral relativism himself, would really dispute that.

As for Beauchamp's worries about the "uniqueness" of an African American perspective on bioethics, I agree that the elements I have mentioned are in no way unique to African Americans. Nor do I know or claim that they are widespread. My claim is that a stance characterized and constituted by them may therein be meaningfully informed by features widespread among African Americans and shaped by experiences many of us have had because we are African American. So, of course, the perspective I sketched is only "contingently and historically" linked to African Americans, as Beauchamp says. To imagine it to be ours necessarily or ahistorically would be absurd.

Third, I ought to add a few remarks on the political theorist Amy Gutmann's critique of my view of culture. Amy Gutmann, "Responding to Racial Injustice," in *Color Conscious: The Political Morality of Race*, ed. K. Anthony Appiah and Amy Gutmann (Princeton, NJ: Princeton University Press, 1996), 175–77, n. 79. Gutmann faults me for having held any culture to be that of some community, whose members must as such be unified around some shared projects. I suspect that Gutmann is correct in that a cultural group can be understood more broadly than I did and that I overstated the commonality needed. Indeed, I am more skeptical today of the very claim that the world contains such diversity of distinct cultural groups. Let me say only that I do not mean to endorse the "tightly scripted" group identities that rightly worry Appiah and to which Gutmann wrongly ties me. Quite the contrary. I doubt we do well to think of people as possessing cultural (or racial) identities at all (either in place of or addition to racial membership), let alone ones to which they should feel obliged to be loyal or on whose basis they should appraise others' racial "authenticity." See my following critical discussion of identity, and authenticity, its usual companion. Griffith's contribution to this volume takes a more sympathetic approach to this way of speaking and thinking. After all, not every group to which someone belongs gives her an identity, and more needs to be said by the proponent of "social identities" to show that and, furthermore, why membership in a cultural or racial group should be thought to do so. For discussions focused on my doubts about ethnic identity, specifically, Latina/o identity, see J. Garcia, "Racial and Ethnic Identity?" in *Race or Ethnicity? Black and Latino Identity*, ed. J. J. E. Gracia (Ithaca, NY: Cornell University Press, forthcoming). This article also raises difficulties about scalar and comparative ethnoracial discourse— "How Black are you?" "She's not very or really Latina," "He's not Black enough," and so forth. In J. L. A. Garcia, "Three Scalarities: Racialization, Racism, and Race," *Theory & Research in Education* 1, no. 3 (2003): 283–302, I develop these criticisms further and direct them also against viewpoints couched in the rubric of racial authenticity.

19. Patricia King's contribution to this volume helpfully treats this issue in greater detail. See especially her discussion of the new drug BiDil, recently tested for exclusive use in treating of heart problems in African Americans, among whom its use seems to have been effective after it was found to have efficacy on white patients. The early journalistic treatment in Carolyn Johnson, "Should Medicine Be Colorblind?" *Boston Globe*, August 24, 2004, pp. C1, C4, offers a fuller discussion of some of the controversy over "look[ing] to race as a rough marker for underlying genetic differences." Johnson quotes lawyer and bioethicist Jonathan Kahn as holding that federal approval of the drug's use for African American, but not white, patients would "have the federal government giving . . . its stamp of approval to using race as a biological category. . . . To my mind, that's the road to hell being paved with good intentions." (On the question of possible racial distinctiveness of congestive heart failure, see R. L. Scott, "Is Heart Failure in African Americans a Distinct Entity?" *Congestive Heart Failure* 9 [2003]: 193–96. For more by the person whose argument is shaping the debate on racialized medical research and prescription, see Jonathan Kahn, "How a Drug Becomes 'Ethnic,' " *Yale Journal of Health Policy, Law, and Ethics* 4 [2004]: 1–46.) Other thinkers interviewed or discussed in Johnson's article express concern lest such use divert attention from socioeconomic factors in disease and in health disparities between races.

20. Appiah, "Race, Culture, and Identity," 30–105.

21. Naomi Zack, *Philosophy of Science and Race* (New York: Routledge, 2002).

22. Joshua Glasgow, "On the New Biology of Race," *Journal of Philosophy* 100 (2003): 456–74.

23. Lucius Outlaw, *On Race and Philosophy* (New York: Routledge, 1996).

24. Philip Kitcher, "Race, Ethnicity, Biology, Culture," in *Racism*, ed. Leonard Harris (Amherst, NY: Humanity Press, 1999), 87–117.

25. Michael Hardimon, "The Ordinary Concept of Race," *Journal of Philosophy* 100 (2003): 437–55.

26. David Wasserman, "Species and Races, Chimeras, and Multiracial People," *American Journal of Bioethics* 3 (2003): 13a–15a.

27. Paul Taylor, "Pragmatism and Race," in *Pragmatism and the Problem of Race*, ed. William E. Lawson and Donald F. Koch (Bloomington: Indiana University Press, 2004), 162–76.

28. Thomas Shelby, "Foundations of Black Solidarity," *Ethics* 112 (2002): 231–66.

29. David Goldstein and Huntington Willard, "Race and the Genome," *Boston Globe*, January 17, 2005, p. A11.

30. Wheelwright reports that representatives of Nitromed, which makes BiDil, pledged at a summer 2004 meeting of the National Medical Association to continue looking for underlying genetic markers while they also specially market the drug to African Americans. Jeff Wheelwright, "Human, Study Thyself," *Discover* (March 2005): 39–44. Having interviewed the influential black geneticist Georgia Dunston, Wheelwright also notes that she deems this commitment necessary but minimal. He quotes her: "You have to characterize the individuals in the [targeted racial] group. . . . What about those who didn't respond [positively to treatment]? The [racial] group just tells us where to drop the net, but we can't stop there, and target the group [for treatment] without the [underlying causal] mechanism known." Wheelwright, "Human," 43–44. His discussion with Dunston reveals the delicate balancing act involved in responsibly addressing race in medical research. Dunston is known for insisting both that medical researchers need to make more vigorous efforts to include black subjects if their results are to be generalizable and also that racial targeting of treatments is scientifically dubious. She sees no contradiction in this pair of positions, though they pull in different directions on medicine's utilizing racial categories. She is probably correct about that, and though I'm not expert in any medical science, each of her two positions here seems persuasive.

31. The readings listed at the end include a number of studies of these disparities. The most important and extensive of these is probably the monumental two-volume work by W. Michael Byrd and Linda A. Clayton, *An American Health Dilemma* (New York: Routledge, 2000–2002).

32. See Byrd and Clayton, *American Health Dilemma*, for one of many discussions of such disparities.

33. My discussion here follows and draws on Lawrence A. Blum, "Systemic and Individual Racism, Racialization, and Antiracist Education," *Theory Research in Education* 2 (March 2004): 49–74, for some of its questions. See esp. p. 53.

34. For an approach like this, see James P. Sterba, *The Demands of Justice* (Notre Dame, IN: University of Notre Dame Press, 1980).

35. Dula's contribution to this volume critically discusses a very different assessment of the ethics of the Tuskegee study, one offered by politically conservative investigators.
36. See Howard McGary, "Distrust, Social Justice, and Health Care," *Mt. Sinai Journal of Medicine* 66 (1999): 236–40.
37. For more on this, see Michael Sandel, "The Case Against Perfection," *Atlantic Monthly* (April 2004): 50–62, and President's Council on Bioethics, *Beyond Therapy: Biotechnology and the Pursuit of Happiness* (New York: Regan Books, 2003). My questions in this section are heavily influenced by both these reflections.

CHAPTER 2

The Moral Weight
of Culture in Ethics

Segun Gbadegesin

S O C I A L anthropology once had to nurse the self-inflicted wound of its characterization as a discipline that is insensitive to the values and identities of other cultures. Seeing non-Western cultures through the prism of a chauvinistic Western male, and judging the modes of life of others by Western standards, earned some pioneer social anthropologists and their political associates (who assumed the "burden of the White Man") the unenviable title of cultural imperialists.[1] With a new orientation, however, anthropology has corrected the mistakes of its pioneers. This new orientation, roundly commended across non-Western cultures, especially in Africa by the apostles of Negritude, was the harbinger of cultural pluralism.[2] Stepping away from an arrogant ethnocentrism, anthropologists started to sing the praises of cultural diversity. They pointed to the distinctiveness of African cultural forms and the need to preserve them. They accepted the idea that each culture has something to offer to the "civilization of the universal," as Senghor would later put it.[3] But the matter became more complex. For there soon began a shift from "cultures differ, and each culture deserves respect" to "morality differs from culture to culture, and no one culture has the right to impose its own moral views on others." Recent anthropology thus gave birth to ethical relativism.[4] With this new development, many of those who had welcomed the discipline's recognition of the plurality of cultures began to worry about the relativistic inference drawn from its thesis. Does morality differ from culture to culture? And what exactly does this mean?

The central claim of relativism is that morality differs across cultures. This is ambiguous. It could mean that moral beliefs differ, in which case it is true. The moral belief of a traditional Yoruba about premarital sex between a prospective husband and wife is influenced by Yoruba customs and tradition. It may or may not differ from that of a tradition-oriented American about the same practice, depending on the similarities between the customs and traditions of the two peoples. Moral beliefs arise from various sources: custom, parents, peers, religion, school, and so on. Therefore, if what "morality differs across cultures" means is that moral beliefs differ, then there is some truth to the matter. It is equally true that moral rules that arise from the application of those moral beliefs differ. Thus a society that holds the moral belief that "lying under pressure is all right" would have no moral rule against the practice.

For its part, universalism insists that to make sense of these so-called differences we need to address our minds to a deeper question: What is the rationale for these moral beliefs? How do the indigenes justify them? One response might be that this thinking is what we inherited from our forebears, which raises the further question, "What could have been the rationale our forebears had for these moral beliefs?" Pressed further, it may soon become clear that we are looking for moral principles that serve as rationale and justification for the moral beliefs. Surely the masses may not have addressed this question before. But it is more than likely that at least some of the thinkers among them would come up with an answer to the question of the rationale or justification for the moral beliefs they hold. Such answers, to our surprise, may coincide with the answers provided by those with different or opposing moral beliefs. The universalist suggests that if we focus on the circumstances that give rise to different moral beliefs, we may have a better understanding of what is going on. Thus the group that believes in the rightness of killing aged parents may see it as a pious obligation that must be discharged in their old age, in view of the "miseries" associated with advanced age and the perceived need to relieve their aged ones of those miseries. Before we see this as an irreconcilable difference in the morality of different cultures, we ought to at least explore the reason for the "differences." Ethical relativism fails to engage in such an exploration.

Of course, universalism is conscious of the possibility that, after we have explored the basis of the various moral beliefs in the principles, there are still differences at the *level of* principles. Disagreements about principles may be fundamental and therefore irreconcilable. However, the fact of such a disagreement cannot be a victory for ethical relativism, because disagreements about principles also occur within specific individual cultures as much as between cultures. Individuals in a particular culture may be right or wrong about the ethical thing to do in specific situations. If they are right, it is not because the culture approves of what they say or do. By the same token, if they are wrong, it is not because the culture disapproves of what they say or do. The moral rightness or wrongness of a person's conduct is independent of the cultural pronouncements therein. Therefore, for the universalist, just the fact of disagreement would not support the relativist inference from differences in cultural moral beliefs to irreconcilable differences in morality across cultures.

My goal here is to address a question not unrelated to the dispute between the relativist and the universalist: What is the moral weight of culture in ethics? It is a complex question that requires us to raise several questions. We need an account of what ethics is, or at least an account of what ethics we have in mind. For instance, how is "moral" different from "ethics" such that the question of the "moral" weight of an X in "ethics" makes sense? Can we also ask for the "ethical" weight of an X in "ethics"? Why not also ask for the moral weight of ethics in culture? We also need an account of what culture is and how it is related, if at all, to morality and/or ethics. I start with the latter question.

What Is Culture?

I identify two senses of culture, one of which is relevant to our topic. In one sense, culture is an activity, specifically a "tending activity," in which sense it is opposed to nature, which is supposedly its raw material for tending. This is the sense in which we talk of a cultured person. It is on this sense of culture that Alain Locke focuses our attention when he declares that "the highest intellectual duty is the duty to be cultured."[5] Elaborating further, Locke observes, "[Culture is] the capacity for understanding the best and most representative forms of human expression, and of expressing oneself, if not in similar creativeness, at least in appreciative reactions and in progressively responsive refinement of tastes and interests."[6] Culture here "suggests a dialectic between the artificial and the natural, what we do to the world and what the world does to us," as Terry Eagleton puts it.[7] A cultured person is a refined person, one who has been worked upon by culture and liberated from nature. But this also suggests that culture is a product of nature, even as it also changes nature. Here culture takes the sense of civilization. What is interesting about this sense of culture is that it allows us to pose an evaluative question of culture. If culture is tending natural growth, we may ask if the tending is done right. After all, in any particular case of tending, the activity and its outcome may be evaluated. Furthermore, culture here lends itself to a double meaning: what *is* and what *ought to be*, where the standard for what ought to be can be anything from morality to aesthetics.

The abovementioned sense of culture apparently conflicts with, or at least is different from, the sense in which it features in contemporary social anthropology. In this sense, popularized by E. B. Tylor, culture is the complex of values, customs, beliefs, and practices that constitute the way of life of a specific group. For Tylor, this complex includes "knowledge, belief, art, *morals*, law, custom, and any other capabilities and habits acquired by man as a member of society."[8] Eagleton reminds us that this sense of the concept is traceable to Herder and the German Idealists. If Enlightenment is identifiable with the first sense, culture there has some appeal to universalism. But in the Herderian sense, culture "means not some grand, unilinear narrative of universal humanity, but a diversity of specific life-forms, each with its own peculiar laws of evolution."[9] If the first sense (culture as tending; as civilization) is universalizable, it is only in the sense that European ideals of "tending" and "civility" can be transported to the whole world; at least, this is how Eurocentrists want it understood. It is partly in revolt against this that Herder's formulation makes sense. "He is out to oppose the Eurocentrism of culture-as-universal-civilization with the claims of those 'of all the quarters of the globe' who have not lived and perished for the dubious honor of having their posterity made happy by a speciously superior European culture."[10] Here, culture becomes the opposite of civility. Indeed, to be civilized in the "European" sense becomes the antithesis of culture or of being cultured, because culture in that sense of "civilization" takes the form of plundering other lands and life forms, a barbaric pursuit. Culture in the Herderian sense is primitive, organic, and authentic from this point of view. It is also sympathetic to the claim that all cultures are equal. For if there is no basis for evaluating life forms as superior or inferior, good or bad, it follows that every life form is equal and is as good as another. It would also follow that it is wrong to elevate one life form over another, and every life form would then seem to have equal moral weight. This argument elides a problem. The assertion that every life form is good fails to consider that there are obviously inconsistent life forms: the life form of the enslaved versus the life form of the slave master. If each life form is good to its practitioner, does it follow that they are equally good to all? But how do we address this question without denying that every life form has some moral weight as culture, especially if *morals* are a component of culture, as the foregoing Tylorian definition suggests.

What Is Ethics?

The question of whether every life form has an equal moral weight leads us to the question, "What is ethics?" I want to approach this question by exploring two recent contributions. In his presidential address to the first annual meeting of the central division (formerly western division) of the American Philosophical Association on May 2, 1986, Professor Marcus G. Singer drew a distinction between three concepts of morality: positive or customary or conventional morality (customary morality, for clarity), personal morality, and rational morality. Customary morality is the accepted morality of a group or culture. It refers to "the standards that most members of the group normally follow or profess to follow or believe they follow or think they should follow, in their own conduct and in their criticism of their own conduct and the conduct and character of others."[11] It consists of rules and principles, which members appeal to in making their judgment of their conduct and of others, and these rules are taught to the young ones and enforced by social pressure. Personal morality, according to Singer, "consists of one's own ideas of right and wrong, derived from principles, rules and beliefs, which sometimes do guide one's own conduct and/or one's judgment of others' conduct."[12] The personal morality of an individual does not necessarily conform to the customary morality of the group to which she or he belongs. This is why an individual may criticize the morality of her group and why a customary morality may be reformed on the basis of a generalized critique from its members. Finally, Singer identifies a third form of morality, rational morality, which is "a presupposition of any criticism of positive morality, past or present" and is presupposed in our critical moral judgments, those based or thought to be based on reason.[13] When we judge the customary morality of our group as inadequate on the basis of our personal morality, we are in fact appealing to the court of rational morality whose standard is reason. Rational morality, then, "is the basis for all fundamental criticism of social institutions, including the institution of positive morality."[14]

The usefulness of the foregoing distinctions should not be overlooked. Every society or culture has the three forms or types of morality. Every society has at least a customary morality. Every person in every society has a personal morality. By the same token, every society, through its members, appeals to rational morality when they make critical judgment of others or change their minds regarding a moral belief or practice. The task is to sort out the principles and rules of rational morality and differentiate them from the rules and principles of customary morality. One important difference is that, unlike the rules and principles of rational morality, the rules and principles of customary morality (in any society) are based on or derived from ideas of life as lived in the society. With the benefit of hindsight, however, members usually come to realize that much of such ideas is based on inadequate (sometimes, mythical) thinking or on fear and prejudice.[15] Rational morality is ethics in the philosophical sense, and it is this sense that I want to use to address the question of the moral weight of culture in ethics. The reason for this is clarified by the second approach that is relevant to my purpose here.

In *Ethical Life: The Past and Present of Ethical Cultures*, Harry Redner distinguishes between ethos and ethics. An ethos is "that portion of the culture of a society concerned with everything to do with conduct and behavior and, in general, with what can be called the style of life."[16] Other forms of life include technique and representation. A civil ethos is attached to a civilization as its product. But it is a preethical aspect of the civilization because it lacks "self-criticism, either philosophically or historically."[17] It is also a precritical ethos. This does not prevent civilizations from carrying on as if their civil ethos is the mark of humanity, leading to clashes between them. (Here civilization is interchangeable with culture in the sense that it is a form of life.)

In spite of such conflicts, civilizations have in common "four fundamental institutions of civility, those associated with the temple (the seat of religion), the court (the symbolic center of authority and power), the city (the civic arena for citizens to pursue their ways of life), and the state (the practical apparatus of rule and administration or officialdom)."[18] Each of these develops its ethos. Redner then argues that ethics arises from a preexisting civil ethos, in the context of a civilization that has gone through a historical development or cultural transformation. An ethic arises out of a preexisting civilized ethos "when the traditionally accepted and unquestioned codes of civility—the divinely-sanctioned laws, the mores and customs, the manners, the conventional duties, the praise-worthy virtues—become subject to higher critical standards and are systematically revised."[19] The "critical standards" are, in turn, based on "a reformulated worldview involving a new transcendent conception of Truth or Reality and a new sense of community."[20] Here, ethics is critical, or refined, ethos.

Though it is not Redner's conclusion, it seems we can infer that ethics as critical or refined ethos is rational morality in Singer's sense. Redner does not reach this conclusion, because he wants to preserve the autonomy of each "ethical culture" or "ethical civilization." For him, the cultural transformation that changes or converts "ethos" into "ethics" is still internal to each civilization and may preserve the differences between the civilizations. For instance, the four types of ethics he identifies include Western and Eastern moralities, which are based on a conception of a higher power and on transcendent principles of religion; civic ethics, which are based on a conception of a higher order (*cosmos, nomos, logos, dike*); ethics of duty, which are based on a system of official laws; and ethics of honor or chivalry. Each of these is derived from a preexisting civilized ethos or forms of civility, namely, the temple/church, city, court, and state, respectively. And even in their developed ethical forms, there is no reason to expect that they might share norms or principles. For ethics is one and many. It is many because there are different ethical traditions that do not merge, hence the clashes between them. But ethics is also one because all ethics have certain features in common: they are all formulated on the basis of the notions of transcendent reality, either a supreme Power or Order that were developed in association with "the religions and philosophies associated with the earliest saviors and sages of world history."[21] Conversely, rational morality presupposes a congruence of principles derived from reason.

In spite of this apparent difference between the two approaches, Redner's analysis leaves open the possibility of a third level of ethical discourse (the first being precritical ethos and the second critical ethics), that is, the level of universal rational ethics. At this level, ethics results from a *common agreement* on core fundamental principles based on or derived from reason. One argument against this is the existence of competing ethical theories.

But this reality does not negate the prospect of rational agreement on fundamental principles. There is no ethical theory that rejects the principle "any action that causes unnecessary pain is morally wrong." There is also no reason to think that this cannot be agreed to across cultures. It has been suggested by relativists that there could still be disputes over what constitutes an unnecessary pain. However, in my judgment, relativists have spilled an undue amount of ink over this matter, which can be rationally resolved by appeal to common sense. Therefore, if the third level of ethical discourse is attainable, Redner's ethics and Singer's rational morality can come to an agreement, and we can then raise the question of the moral weight of culture (understood as a form of life) in ethics (understood as rational morality). In any case, for both Redner and Singer, it is safe to infer that ethics is a cultural practice: this is clear in the case of Redner. It seems also clear in the case of Singer, for whom ethics is the outcome of rational reflections on the moral institution, where the moral institution is an integral part of culture. Paraphrasing Amilcar Cabral, we may say that ethics is an act of culture.[22]

What, If Anything, Is the Role of Ethics in Culture?

In both conceptions, ethics has a significant role to play in culture. As rational morality, it serves as the conscience of culture through its critique of cultural practices, thus making cultural progress possible. As a developed ethical form from preexisting civil ethos, ethics in Redner's sense also serves as the conscience of the particular civilization. It probes its standards, subjects them to higher critical standards, and systematically revises them. Importantly, no culture is completely homogeneous or monolithic. There are segments and hybrids. Thus, within an otherwise "whole way of life" may be several "quasi-independent ways of lives." In such a situation, ethics as rational morality serves the purpose of filtering through the maze of life forms and reconciling them with its appeal to critical standards. Such an approach requires humility and tolerance. If it is assumed that each life form, as such, has some moral legitimacy, then any critical standard that rational morality would bring to bear on it must proceed with the mind-set of a learner, not of a teacher. The idea is that the culture has something to teach us as outsiders, and we are prepared to learn. In the process, we confront some aspects of it that challenge our moral sensibilities. If it is based on a morality that is not quite similar to ours, we have to ask for education. Perhaps it will become clear, or if it does not, perhaps we can discuss on the conflicting moralities and come to an agreement. In many cases, dialogue reveals acceptable agreement, if not truth, and that is good enough.

What Is the Moral Weight of Culture in Ethics?

The answer to the question "What is the moral weight of culture in ethics?" may provide an anchor for relativism. It seems to me that the moral weight of culture in ethics is *relative* to the cultural practice in question and its effect on human flourishing. The core of morality is the promotion of human flourishing, and therefore a critical standard for evaluating a civil ethos is the extent to which it promotes or negates human flourishing. If a cultural practice truly enhances human flourishing, the moral weight of the culture is heavy, and it deserves careful attention. If, alternatively, a cultural practice negates or retards human flourishing, the moral weight of the culture is very light, and may indeed be nil.

Again, relativism may raise the issue of the alleged variation of ideas of human flourishing across cultures. A short answer to this allegation is that it misconstrues the notion of human flourishing because the notion does not lend itself to a *cultural* determination as such. Human flourishing is *individual* human flourishing, and this requires an individual to be able to do certain things and be a certain kind of person. An individual flourishes when he or she is not hampered not only from satisfying his or her basic needs but also from *aspiring* to higher levels of attainment. An individual flourishes when he or she is capable of participating in the affairs of the community as a free person with human dignity. Even if we grant the influence of culture on conceptions of human flourishing, it does not follow that cultures cannot come to an agreement on a thin conception of human flourishing that can serve as a principle of adjudication.

Thus I agree with Thomas Pogge that "though disagreements about what human flourishing consists in may prove ineradicable, it may well be possible to bypass them by agreeing that nutrition, clothing, shelter, and certain basic freedoms, as well as social interaction, education, and participation, are important means to it—means which just social institutions must secure for all."[23] This eliminates certain practices, for instance, the practice of human sacrifice. Clearly, the practice negates the flourishing of the individual victim, and it has no redeeming social value. If the belief is that the sacrifice would pacify the gods and bring the much needed rainfall, we know that it is misplaced, and it is useless to defend the belief on the ground that it works for the people because it does not. Moreover, it does a disservice to the common humanity that we lay claim to by suggesting that the people are the best judge in that situation.

If, however, a cultural practice has a negative impact on individual human flourishing and it has a redeeming social value, say, in the survival of the society, then the moral weight of the culture is not inconsequential. An example here is the case of a "just" war, if war can be described as a cultural practice. In this case, however, the sacrifice it entails for individuals must be distributed fairly across the social spectrum. A cultural practice is not self-justifying. Appealing to the concept of human flourishing, we may now revisit and revise the argument for the relativity or equality of life forms, which we encountered earlier. We must now observe that every life form/ cultural practice deserves a prima facie equal consideration. But where there is a conflict in the practices of life forms/cultural practices, we must appeal to a principle of adjudication. An adequate principle of adjudication is the principle of human flourishing. Therefore, a life form/cultural practice that negates human flourishing does not deserve equal consideration. I follow this reasoning in the subsequent discussion of some cases in cross-cultural bioethics.

Cultural Differences in Health Care: Differences in Ethics of Health Care across Cultures

There is a need to make a distinction between cultural differences in health care and differences in ethics of health care across cultures. By the former, I mean differences in how particular cultures approach health care. Thus, in many traditional societies, whether in Africa, Asia, or the Caribbean, there is still a strong belief in the efficacy of spiritual healing. This is also true of religious communities. Christians, especially those of the fundamentalist or evangelical sort, put a lot of faith in the power of prayer, and the Jehovah's Witnesses' rejection of blood transfusion points to another dimension of the issue. In all of these cases, one may justifiably conclude that there are cultural differences in our approaches to health care. Such differences normally raise ethical questions, that is, questions about the moral acceptability of some approaches vis-à-vis others, or questions about the morally acceptable way to resolve moral problems that come up in the application of one approach or another. This is the focus of what I refer to as the ethics of health care. For instance, if the diviner's verdict is that the sickness of the child is due to the mischief of the witch, and that for the child to get better, the witch has to be confronted, then what ethical problem is raised by this approach, and how do we approach its resolution? Should we worry about the subjective nature of the verdict? Should we be bothered about false accusation? Should we even worry that the sick child may not get better even after the confrontation with the witch? These are ethical issues about this particular cultural approach to health care, and these questions may get answered in different ways. How they are answered is a reflection of the *moral perception* of each group or culture. The distinctive aspect of these questions, and the way they are answered in different cultures, is that those answers are not sacrosanct, precisely because moral perceptions are not sacrosanct. They may be challenged, modified, or dropped, and that is what the ethics of health care practices is about, its focus being to come up with ethically sound answers.

While the first set of issues (cultural differences in health care) comes up regularly in the literature, the second set (differences in the ethics of health care across cultures) is either ignored, underemphasized, or collapsed into the first. Or, in the worst case, the first set of issues is taken as the ethical differences. Thus, if traditional Africans insist on dealing with a child's health condition by identifying a witch as the culprit, it is immediately concluded that it is within their ethics, and no one can do or say anything about it. Or we identify the practice of decision making that involves an extended family as the typical African approach—a cultural practice, which differs from the Euro-American practice—and then we suggest that it marks a difference in the ethics of health care between the two cultures. There is a tendency, as Richard Lieban rightly noted, "to view the ethical aspects of health care in other cultures as cultural givens and to neglect ways in which they may relate to moral questions and ambiguities."[24] In the literature, cultural differences get identified as ethical differences, and cultural particularity is taken to entail ethical relativism. What is needed is a critical analysis of the moral problems and issues raised by culturally specific medical actions as they occur in different cultures, especially non-Western cultural settings.

The questions "How ought we to act?" or "How ought our society to be organized?" are at the heart of all social or cultural concerns that agitate the minds of the founders of societies from Africa to the West. These are ethical questions. The way the societies answer these questions may be dictated by the realities they confront at one particular time. Because particular times are not *eternally* privileged, one should expect that as circumstances change, the answers they generate will also change. But more to the point, one should expect that given the realities they face at any one point in time, founders of societies might not have the best answers to the ethical questions they try to address. In such situations, those answers cannot enjoy the sanctity of an eternal truth. This is to suggest that individuals, even those who are guardians of cultural ethos, may be wrong about some moral claims or prescriptions. Yet what is important is to get it right, to have the right answer to the moral questions that the culture faces. What the foregoing observation suggests is that rather than privilege cultural practices without question, we should address the prior concerns and questions to which those practices provide answers, and then ask whether they are the right kinds of answers given the circumstances. In other words, cultural practices are answers (even if implicitly formulated) to ethical questions about how we ought to act and how our society ought to be organized. This does not contradict the earlier claim that ethics is a cultural practice. It is a cultural practice that yields outcomes that may also be critically assessed in the light of other practices. Rationality is as much a cultural practice as ethics. When we approach the matter in this way, we would begin to appreciate the interplay and complexity of ethics and culture in general, and the ethics of health care and health care practices across cultures in particular. In what follows, I review some cases of different health care practices, with a view to showing the ethical issues they raise even as they hide behind the façade of culture.

Case 1: The Mananambal (Folk Healers) of the Cebuano Areas of the Philippines

In "Medical Anthropology and the Comparative Study of Medical Ethics," Richard Lieban reports that the mananambal are folk healers and that the "morality of a *mananambal* is considered to have a vital bearing on his own well-being and on his effectiveness as a healer."[25] If he does not perform his moral obligations, he may become sick or insane, or he may lose his healing power and his prestige and livelihood. He has a moral duty to help his clients and to be truthful. In this society, however, and given the perception that the healer is spiritually endowed, there is power relation between the healer and the patient, the former being considered as superior. An important consequence is that what features in the ethics of health care in the West— privacy and confidentiality—may be illusive here. Lieban gave the example of a patient who was told in front of other patients by her mananambal that she was not a virgin. Lieban adds, significantly, that the lady "had never returned (to the healer) and once had crossed the street to avoid him."[26] We may see this as an example of a different practice and then raise ethical questions about it. Is it morally right? The tendency in anthropological discourse, however, is to see it as the practice of the people, the moral acceptability of which should not be the concern of outsiders. Yet the further question can be raised if it is obvious from this example whether the behavior of the healer was acceptable to the insiders. How did the lady see it? Why did she not return? Was it because she felt ashamed of her action? Was it because she was embarrassed in front of everybody? Should not such feelings make a difference from an ethical point of view? Would the matter be different if the healer had told her his verdict in private? And in terms of the effectiveness of the system, without the practice of respect for privacy, would the system be able to sustain itself? These are legitimate questions, and it makes sense to suggest that people internal to the system may be asking these questions as well. The lady in this case presumably was not persuaded that the mananambal did the right thing.

Lieban points to this case as an example of the difference in the ethics of health care. I see it as an example of a difference in health care practices, which raises ethical questions, some of which I raised earlier, especially about the importance of privacy. This practice of the mananambal needs to be critically analyzed and appraised. One of the concerns of the mananambal is the consequence of not being truthful. If the healer fails to tell the truth as he sees it, there is the fear that he may suffer some misfortune, including sickness or loss of healing power. So it is clear that the interest of the healer is also at stake in this matter. But the question is, is there a more decent way of letting the patient know about the verdict of the gods on her "waywardness"? Perhaps there is a more altruistic rationale for the practice. If the truth is told in public, it may have a deterrent effect on the other patients around, and by extension on the rest of the population, who are bound to hear the gossip. By the same token, this anticipated "positive" consequence could be weighed against the possible negative outcome of the practice. Many "wayward" young women may avoid going to the healer; this may affect his own popularity and income, and more importantly, it may affect the health care of the people, if the healer is in fact effective in this area. Obviously, these are considerations of utility or expediency. Is there a particular consideration that speaks to the humanity of the patient that can be invoked against the practice of public exposure of a patient by the healer? The fact of the humanity of the patient is enough to suggest a different approach. Like the rest of us, the young woman has feelings: she could feel shame, she could be devastated by open humiliation, she could feel disgraced. The evidence that all these feelings were experienced by the lady is supplied in Lieban's narrative of the case: she never returned to the healer. These feelings of shame, disgrace, and humiliation are universal and could be bases for appraising the practice of the mananambal. And in the event that they respond that these feelings don't count or are irrelevant to appraising their practice, we would, contrary to relativism, have to say that they are mistaken.

Case 2: Veracity and Disclosure

Sticking to the fieldwork of Lieban among the Cebuano people, there is another report that focuses on veracity and disclosure. The cultural belief of the people in sorcery and witchcraft is similar to many traditional African peoples. For Lieban, the ethical issue here is disclosure and veracity: When is it morally acceptable to disclose information to a patient about the cause of her illness? Is it right to tell the patient that a sorcerer is responsible for her condition, even when the mananambal knew that fact? If one does, it may disrupt social relations in the community. If one does not, one violates the rule of disclosure and truth telling. Lieban concludes that, "under these circumstances, the ethics of disclosure has to be viewed in a context wider than the patient's right to medical information and the healer's obligation to provide it."[27]

I see the matter differently. I do not think that we have here a case of differences in ethics, but rather a case of epistemological conflict. In what sense does the mananambal *know* that the *sorcerer* is responsible for the illness of the patient? Surely it is not a "knowledge" that is based on any valid deduction. At best, one could claim that the mananambal believes, based on the common belief of his society, that there are sorcerers and that they are typically credited with the cause of certain types of illness. But such a belief could be, and has often been shown to be, mistaken. Because that is the case, there is no need here to worry about the ethics of disclosure, because what needs to be disclosed is that the mananambal has no knowledge of the cause of the illness. Compare a different scenario: The mananambal discovers that the patient has been poisoned by her co-wife, having listened to the confession of the latter, who released the remainder of the poison to the mananambal, who is then able to test the poison and confirm it as the cause of the patient's illness. The mananambal then becomes concerned about the consequence of his disclosing the cause of illness to the patient because of the relationship between the perpetrator of the act and the victim. Unlike the previous example, here we have a clear case of an ethical dilemma, which, incidentally, is not different from its occurrence in Western bioethics and may therefore be approached in the same way.

Case 3: Woman Wants Husband's Approval for ER Admission

A traditional Yoruba woman registers at an antenatal clinic. One day after examining her, the physician tells her that her blood pressure is high and that she would need to be admitted into the hospital ward. Because her husband and relations are not there with her, the woman volunteers to consult with her husband about the matter. The physician wonders whether this is necessary, because it is the woman's health and that of her fetus at stake.

Does this suggest a moral dilemma for the physician? Does it suggest a fundamental difference in the ethics of informed consent between the Western-trained physician and the woman? I do not see any moral dilemma posed by this episode. The woman is within her right to consult with anybody before consenting to any form of treatment, and she has chosen to exercise that right.

Suppose that, after consultation, she decides not to go in to the hospital. Possible interpretations could be that the husband has ordered her not to, or it may be that after listening to the analysis of the consequences of her admission, the woman decides against admission. If the former, there is a concern that such a thing cannot happen in the West, and this suggests a difference in ethics. It is, however, a question of what empirical evidence one has for determining the motivating force behind the woman's decision. Assume that we have evidence that the woman has been so ordered by her husband and that she has accordingly obeyed the order. What questions does this raise, if any? For me, it does not then mean that an ethical appraisal of the situation from an objective point of view is not in order. This would especially make sense if it is not the case that other women have been so imposed upon by their husbands. But even if it is a common practice, the question "Is it right?" is still not out of place. The principle here, again, is that what is a common cultural practice (imposition on wives by their husbands) could be appraised from an ethical point of view: Is it right? This appraisal is especially necessary because those non-Western societies also deal with ethical issues within their cultures.

What, for instance, would a traditional healer do if such a situation arises that he has to treat a pregnant woman for an illness? The healer would inform the woman about her ailment and what needs to be done about it. The healer would then ask her to discuss the matter with her husband, and if he has any questions, he should come and see the healer. The healer would discuss the matter with the man on a man-to-man basis, addressing any questions the man may have. The woman is not left out of the picture, because it is after the woman has agreed to the need for the treatment that the husband is brought in. It is not common under that circumstance for the husband to refuse. If he does, it would be understood by the woman (and her relations) that he does not take an interest in her health. Many a woman has used that as a reason for divorce, at least in traditional Yoruba society. The consultation with the husband is in part predicated on the fact that the husband has responsibility to take care of his wife and to pay the necessary fees to the healer. Does this suggest a different account of informed consent? Is it unusual for family members in the West to hold consultations with one another on a course of treatment prescribed by a physician? From all accounts, including the recommendations in the various guidelines, it is not unusual, and physicians do recommend it, though there may be less degree of regularity in its occurrence in the West.

Case 4: Mother Is Daughter's Surrogate

It pays to examine another familiar scenario in traditional health care practice. An adult daughter, Laide, is seriously ill. Her mother, Sade, goes to consult the healer-diviner on behalf of Laide, the daughter. By the time that Sade gets to the diviner, other clients are waiting to see him. Sade takes her place on the queue. When it is her turn, she presents her problem to the healer by whispering to the divination chain. The healer takes the chain and consults with the oracle, chants some verses of the corpus until he strikes at Sade's problem: illness in the family. The healer tells Sade what to do—offer sacrifice to the gods and give some herbal medicine, which he supplied, to Laide. Later the healer visits Laide in Sade's presence, listens to her complaints, and gives her more herbal remedies.

It would appear that this is a different world entirely. At least, it is not a world that takes seriously the issue of patient autonomy, privacy, and confidentiality. Before we draw this kind of inference, it should be helpful to understand what is going on in this episode. First, it is clear that this is a typical occurrence in traditional African health care systems. Here, family members assume the role of health care givers, acting as de facto nurses, physician's assistants, medication dispensers, and so on. This is usually in addition to their roles as family members. Therefore the interaction of healers with family members in these settings is similar to physicians' interaction with professionals in the consulting rooms of their various clinics. In the circumstance, the issues of privacy and confidentiality hardly come up. As in this case, the initial contact with the healer is made by the mother who has been taking care of the daughter since the beginning of the latter's illness, which has immobilized her. When the mother can no longer cope because it has become clear that it is not an "ordinary fever," the mother goes to the next step in the health care giver's hierarchy: the healer.

Second, it is important to note that family members, especially parents even of adults, are perceived as metaphysical extensions of their wards. Mother's destiny is tied to daughter's destiny. So it is not strange in this system that the mother is the one that goes to the healer. But is it morally acceptable? The only reason it might not be judged acceptable is that the mother is imposing her will on the daughter and taking advantage of her condition.

Third, there is an expansive notion of self, which makes the patient *see her mother* as part of her extended identity. In the circumstance, there is an enlarged notion of patient autonomy, which includes daughter and mother as one entity. It is a notion that daughter, like mother, internalizes and accepts. For if circumstances were to change and the mother becomes ill, the daughter will play the same role that the mother is now playing. It is a notion that is perhaps different from contemporary Western notion of self, but which is not thereby morally deficient.

Finally, the openness of the consultation with a traditional healer is not an inherent part of the system. It is just that people are not aware of anything wrong with it, having accepted the logic of divination. In any case, it is also understood that a patient can seek privacy. Certainly, it would be a lot better, from a moral point of view, if there were a demarcation between the waiting room and the inner chamber where the healer consults with patients and surrogates, and in many cases, there is such a demarcation. The evidence that the diviner-healer pays attention to privacy is that the patient or her surrogate whispers to the divination chain. She sits closest to the diviner-healer in the consultation room and is within an earshot of the diviner-healer.

Case 5: Different Cultural Beliefs and a Physician's Predicament

Mrs. Ala is a fifty-five-year-old Yoruba who recently migrated to the United States to join her son and daughter-in-law. The woman had a history of high blood pressure. The son is a successful insurance executive, and the daughter-in-law is a nurse. They are both rooted in the Yoruba tradition and in the evangelical Christian faith. About a year after her arrival, Mrs. Ala becomes homesick, and she wants to go back to see her siblings and other grandchildren. Her son is opposed to this, and the old woman's blood pressure becomes unmanageable. One day she goes into a coma but is resuscitated; she then has to be put on life support and is being monitored by a team of physicians. After several months, the physicians inform the son that the mother's situation is irreversible and that the son has to decide if he wants her to continue on life support. For their part, because nothing more could be done, they told him, they would like to remove the life support. The son rejects this advice because, according to him, it is against his culture. The physicians do not want to go against the dictates of a culture they know nothing about. What should they do?

A case like this is the nightmare of Western physicians and ethicists who hate to be accused of cultural arrogance. The question, however, is how can a physician avoid such a charge? First, the veracity of the cultural reference must be ascertained by an independent body or group, and so, an ethics committee, which includes a member of the patient's culture group, is needed to confirm the claim about the cultural belief. In this particular case, it is clear to me that the son may have it wrong. The Yoruba cultural belief in the sanctity of life is refined. There is a prayer against "living just for the sake of living" or "living without really living," which is what existing with devices like life support amounts to for many elderly Yoruba. Therefore Yoruba cultural belief does not support the son. There are cases of aged people who refuse be taken to the hospital and would rather "go home" in peace. Of course, it is also a common occurrence all over the world that a child does not want to let go of a loving parent.

Second, even if it is discovered that the cultural belief of the Yoruba is well represented by the son, that should not be the end of the matter. The question "What then ought we do now?" should still be raised. Suppose, for instance, that *knowing* that she could not ever recover, by keeping the woman on life support, the resources expended on her could be used to help a more hopeful case. It is not clear then that the cultural belief has a more ethical force in this matter. Should we then still privilege the cultural belief? This is a question that an ethics committee should be called upon to address. If the committee decides in favor of withdrawing the life support, a court of law can be called upon to enforce the decision.

Third, as noted earlier, the son may not be covered by appeal to the Yoruba cultural belief, because in that belief, most old and terminally ill people want to make an end quickly and die with dignity, based on the principle of *ikuyajesin*: death is better than living with indignity. However, the son is an evangelical Christian, and he may be transferring his Christian belief into the Yoruba cultural tradition. Even then, the question raised earlier should still apply: Should a religious belief have a moral force if, in fact, the resources could be used to benefit a more hopeful case?

Conclusion: Facts, Questions, and Answers

Where do the foregoing case illustrations lead us? They affirm that the usefulness of anthropological knowledge is that it points out to us at least three basic facts. First, cultural practices that have implications for health (of individuals and community) vary from place to place. Second, health care practices (including conceptions of disease, practitioner-patient relationship, etc.) vary from place to place. Third, moral beliefs about cultural practices that have implications for health and about health care practices vary from place to place. The questions that flow from these facts are essentially two. First, with regard to the variation in cultural practices and health care practices, "What should be the approach of an ethicist?" Second, with regard to the variation in moral beliefs people hold concerning the moral acceptability of such practices, "What should be the approach of an ethicist?"

In my discussion of the cases, I suggested what I believe ought to be the answers to both of these questions. First, an ethicist should try to understand the rationale and meaning of the cultural practices, as well as talk with the community or individual members about the rationale and the health implications of the practices. Many people think—incorrectly, I believe—that once you are able to identify a cultural practice with a people, they, as the practitioners of the culture, must have a vested interest in its perpetuation such that they cannot be persuaded about its potential harm. This is not the case. The killing of twins used to be a cultural practice in some parts of the developing world. It is no longer, and its eradication is appreciated by

those cultures. A cultural practice is not self-justifying. People's moral belief about it is part of what justifies it to them. This leads to the second answer. With respect to moral beliefs, the attitude of an ethicist should again be
first to understand the meaning of the belief, its sources (e.g., is it from tradition or religion?) and the issues it raises (e.g., inconsistencies in its claims,
or negative impact on people's well-being). Then one should be free to make
suggestions for a reassessment of the moral beliefs in the light of the health
implications of the cultural practice that it endorses. Cross-cultural health
care ethics cannot afford to do less.

Notes

1. A famous member of this early school was Lucien Levy-Bruhl. See Lucien Levy-
   Bruhl, *Primitive Mentality* (1923; repr., Boston: Beacon Press, 1966).
2. See Melville J. Herskovits, *Cultural Relativism: Perspective in Cultural Pluralism*
   (New York: Random House, 1972). See also A. R. Radcliffe-Brown, "Science
   and Native Problems: How to Understand Bantu," *Anthropology Today* 2, no. 4
   (1986): 17–21.
3. Leopold Senghor, "Negritude: A Humanism of the Twentieth Century," in *The
   Africa Reader: Independent Africa*, ed. W. Cartey and M. Kilson (New York:
   Random House, 1970), 179–92.
4. Herskovits was one of the defenders of ethical relativism; see *Cultural Rela-
   tivism*. For more on the debate on relativism, see Ruth Benedict, *Patterns of
   Culture* (New York: Mentor Books, 1934); Michel de Montaigne, *The Complete
   Essays of Montaigne*, trans. Donald Frame (Stanford, CA: Stanford University
   Press, 1958); Clifford Geertz, *The Interpretation of Cultures: Selected Essays* (New
   York: Basic Books, 1973). See also Geertz, "Anti Anti-Relativism," *American Anthropologist* 86 (1984): 263–78, and "Of Cannibals and Custom: Montaigne's
   Cultural Relativism," *Anthropology Today* 2, no. 5 (1986): 12–14.
5. Alain Locke, "The Ethics of Culture," in *The Philosophy of Alain Leroy Locke:
   Harlem Renaissance and Beyond*, ed. Leonard Harris (Philadelphia: Temple University Press, 1989), 176.
6. Ibid., 177.
7. Terry Eagleton, *The Idea of Culture* (Malden, MA: Blackwell, 2000), 2.
8. E. B. Tylor, *Primitive Culture* (New York: Harper, 1958). Cited in Eagleton, *Idea
   of Culture*, 34, italics mine.
9. Eagleton, *Idea of Culture*, 12.
10. Ibid.
11. Marcus George Singer, *The Ideal of a Rational Morality* (Presidential address,
    APA Western [Central] Division, 1986), 16.

12. Ibid., 17.
13. Ibid.
14. Ibid., 19.
15. Consider here the many customary moralities of traditional Africans and traditional Europeans: the evil of witchcraft and the practice of witch burning; the evil of twins and the practice of twin killing in Africa, and so on.
16. Harry Redner, *Ethical Life: The Past and Present of Ethical Cultures* (Lanham, MD: Rowman and Littlefield, 2001), 31.
17. Ibid., 34.
18. Ibid., 35.
19. Ibid., 43.
20. Ibid.
21. Ibid., 27.
22. See Amilcar Cabral, "National Liberation and Culture," in *Return to the Source: Selected Speeches of Amilcar Cabral* (New York: Monthly Review Press, 1973).
23. Thomas W. Pogge, "Human Flourishing and Universal Justice," in *Human Flourishing*, vol. 16, ed. Ellen Frankel Paul, Fred D. Miller Jr., and Jeffrey Paul (Cambridge: Cambridge University Press, 1999), 342; Douglass B. Rasmussen, "Human Flourishing and the Appeal to Human Nature," in *Human Flourishing*, vol. 16, 1–43; Martha C. Nussbaum, *Women and Human Development: The Capabilities Approach* (New York: Cambridge University Press, 2000).
24. Richard W. Lieban, "Medical Anthropology and the Comparative Study of Medical Ethics," in *Social Science Perspectives on Medical Ethics*, ed. G. Weisz (Dordrecht, The Netherlands: Kluwer Academic, 1990), 221–39 (quote at p. 221).
25. Ibid., 223.
26. Ibid., 225.
27. Ibid., 226.

CHAPTER 3

Whitewashing Black Health: Lies, Deceptions, Assumptions, and Assertions—and the Disparities Continue

Annette Dula

OVER the last several decades, the federal government and private foundations have focused on the appalling health disparities between racial/ethnic minorities and whites, with their goal being to narrow the health status gap between nonwhites and whites. For example, the 1965 Medicare-Medicaid legislation improved access to health care for African Americans and other poor populations. In 1985, the U.S. Department of Health and Human Services published the *Report of the Secretary's Task Force on Black and Minority Health*, which acknowledged the tragic dilemma of persistent health disparities between whites and minority populations.[1] In 1998, then-president Bill Clinton launched an initiative to reduce and eliminate racial and ethnic disparities by 2010. In 2001, the National Institutes of Health (NIH) established the National Center for Minority Health and Health Disparities (NCMHD), which received an annual budget of $132 million to fight health disparities. In 2002, its budget was increased to $157.8 million, and in 2003 the NIH requested $189 million for NCMHD. Similarly, the Robert Wood Johnson, Kellogg, and Kaiser foundations and the Commonwealth Fund have all taken up the challenge to fight health disparities through research and education.

Despite the many federal and private initiatives aimed at reducing health disparities, despite the numerous academic papers published that raise awareness of the issue, despite new cultural competency requirements of medical schools and continuing education, and despite the changing of African Americans' behaviors, the health disparities continue. In fact, gaps in health status between blacks and whites for some conditions have not changed since 1970, and in some cases may have worsened. For example, in 1970, infant mortality among African Americans was twice that among whites.[2] In 2003, black infant mortality was still twice that of whites. Infant mortality even increased from 2001 for all racial/ethnic groups;[3] tellingly, the increase was statistically significant only for infants of black mothers.[4]

In 1970, deaths due to asthma were about three times higher for blacks than for whites.[5] More than thirty years later, the death rate from asthma for African Americans is still three times the rate for the white population.[6] Several reports have acknowledged that increasing the number of under-represented minority physicians and medical students is an "important strategy in the elimination of racial and ethnic care disparities."[7] Alarmingly, however, the number of black medical graduates declined by 17 percent, from a high of 1,246 in 1998 to 1,034 in 2004. In addition, minorities still account for only 4.2 percent of U.S. medical school faculties.[8]

One is compelled to ask, "Why are health disparities still with us after four decades of serious efforts to eliminate them?" I hypothesize that eliminating health disparities works against the vested interests of powerful political and economic forces. The current conservative agenda, along with a corporate-friendly Congress and White House, promotes and implements policies and practices that are at odds with the task of making health disparities a phenomenon of the past. These forces are not intentionally racist, nor do they aim to worsen disparities between minorities and whites. Rather, more subtly, their practices result in diluting or neutralizing progress toward eliminating health disparities.

My purpose here is to point out how spokespeople for conservative think tanks—fueled by their corporate backers—are constructing narratives that undermine efforts to reduce and eliminate racial health disparities. First, I present five deceptive stories that some groups, individuals, and think tanks are purveying, which dismiss the role of race in the poor health of African Americans. Then I examine three assertions that underlie these stories. And, finally, I discuss how these five stories and their underlying assertions are part of a larger corporate agenda that has bad side effects for the health of African Americans and other poor populations. The stories and assumptions partly explain why the disparities continue despite massive efforts to eliminate them.

Deceptive and Misleading Information— Whitewashing Health Disparities

Story/Lie No. 1: *There is no physician race bias or negative stereotyping in health care.* This is the belief of Sally Satel, a psychiatrist at the American Enterprise Institute.

In March 2002, the Institute of Medicine (IOM) published a landmark study on health disparities.[9] The Institute reviewed more than one hundred previously published peer-reviewed studies and concluded that health disparities are persistent and pervasive and that they are caused in part by negative stereotypes and bias of some physicians.

There were numerous media responses, including that of Sally Satel.[10] Satel says that the IOM's case for prejudice in the health care system is weak and based on dubious research. She believes there is no evidence that supports the accusation of bias in the health care system. Her argument? The IOM uses words such as *some, suggest,* and *may.* When researchers use these words, she advises, it means the data are flimsy. She thinks retrospective studies of the sort used by the IOM are inadequate measures of health disparities.[11]

In her book *PC, MD: How Political Correctness Is Corrupting Medicine,* Satel berates those who advocate for social justice in health care.[12] She scoffs at the notion that racial discrimination can affect physiology, denying the validity of hypertension studies that connect high blood pressure to the stress of racism. She claims that "political correctness" and victim politics contribute to health disparities because they interfere with effective diagnosis and doctoring. As she sees it, disparities are due to problems in access to health care, health education literacy, and personal attitudes and behaviors.

Satel is particularly venomous toward public health academics and bioethicists whom she criticizes for having a social agenda. "Who Needs Medical Ethics?" attacks those who argue that transforming economic conditions will help eliminate health disparities.[13] She has also accused the National Medical Association and the American Medical Association of practicing politically correct medicine and victim politics. She dismisses disparities research as ideologically driven and unable to withstand critical scrutiny. She roundly dismisses the possibility of even unconscious racial bias and racism in medicine, calling it just "media hype."[14]

Satel fails to adequately address the numerous studies—many cited by the IOM report—that connect differential treatment to unconscious bias or stereotyping. Research consistently and persistently shows that African Americans do indeed have problems accessing health care (with which Satel agrees). But we also receive inferior health care as compared with whites. Inequalities in preventive care, diagnostic care, and use of therapeutic procedures have long been reported and analyzed in all prestigious and peer-reviewed medical, policy, law, and social science journals. Denial of a relation between the shameful health status gap and inequalities in care prevents a complete analysis and understanding of the causes of health disparities.

Story/Lie No. 2: *Environmental pollutants do not contribute to health disparities.* This is the view espoused by Christopher Foreman of the Brookings Institution[15] and Michael Gough of the Cato Institute.[16]

For many African Americans, poor health begins long before getting to the doctor's office. It begins in places where we live, work, play, and go to school. Often these places are burdened with an unequal share of exposure to toxic substances from factories and industries—substances that are harmful to health. A growing number of studies show that race is associated with increased levels of exposure to environmental hazards.[17]

"Cancer Alley" is the name given by local residents to a one-hundred-mile corridor along the Mississippi River between Baton Rouge and New Orleans. More than one hundred chemical and oil companies despoil the river. They are disproportionately located near poor and minority communities. Residents in these areas complain of exposure to environmental pollutants spewed by the numerous petrochemical plants. Cases of rare cancers are reported in these communities in numbers above the national average. These communities also complain of clusters of asthma, stillbirths, miscarriages, neurological diseases, and cancers.[18]

Not true, says Christopher Foreman.[19] He maintains that most of the waste sites in communities of color are clean and pose little or no risk to health. The papers and reports that attest to the disproportionate dumping of toxic wastes, the siting of petrochemical companies, and claims of health risks in communities of color are all statistically flawed. He says that the health hazards of dioxin and of hormone disrupters such as polychlorinated biphenyls (PCBs) are unproven. Environmental justice activists, he argues, ought to spend their time encouraging blacks to stop smoking, instead of railing against unfounded health effects of petrochemical facilities in communities of color.

Michael Gough of the Cato Institute agrees with Foreman. He says that Cancer Alley is a big myth.[20] Poor and black Louisianans die from cancer at a higher rate than do people in other states because they are too poor to get medical care, because they smoke at an earlier age, and because they do not eat enough fruits and vegetables. According to Gough, they don't eat fruits and vegetables because they cost too much. Hence it's not the proximity to petrochemicals that causes cancer. On the contrary, the regulation of pesticides is really what contributes to the high numbers of cancer deaths in Louisiana. Pesticide regulation causes food prices to go up; therefore consumption of fruit and vegetables goes down, and the incidence of cancer increases.

Such commentary dismisses the role the environment plays in the poor health of African Americans and other ethnic minorities. It makes light of the fears of people living in dangerously polluted areas over which they have little control because of their economically vulnerable state. Even if sufficient research is lacking to prove a definite connection between cancer and environmental contamination, concerns about environmental health are legitimate and ought to be taken seriously.[21] Dismissal of the health effects of environmental toxins is disingenuous, manipulative, deceptive, and deflects from the goal of reducing health disparities between racial/ethnic minorities and whites.

Whether due to smoking, as Gough maintains,[22] or to environmental contamination, as community activists assert,[23] the cancer death rate in Louisiana is the third highest among the fifty states, after Kentucky and West Virginia.[24] In 2003, the cancer mortality rate per 100,000 people for Louisiana was 228, compared with the national average of 197. Moreover, blacks from Louisiana have a higher incidence of lung, colorectal, and breast cancer than blacks nationally.[25]

Story/Lie No. 3: *The Tuskegee Syphilis Study was not racist,* declares Robert White, an African American medical oncologist based in Silver Spring, Maryland.[26]

In brief, the Tuskegee Syphilis Study (TSS) involved four hundred black syphilitic men and lasted forty years, from 1932 to 1972. Researchers—who wanted to study the natural history of untreated syphilis—told the men that they were being treated for "bad blood"; the research subjects were not informed that they had syphilis, nor did they consent to be in the study. When penicillin became available, it was withheld from them.

In "Unraveling the Tuskegee Syphilis Study of Untreated Syphilis," White concludes that the study was a scientifically and medically valid public health endeavor, and not racist.[27] Unfortunately, he laments, black and white physicians, black people, the media, and researchers—who approach the study with outrage rather than reason—have reconceptualized the study as malpractice on poor and uneducated human guinea pigs. If these people would put away their rage and were more reasonable, he says, we would all see that allegations of racism, exploitation, differential treatment, and denial of state-of-the-art treatment do not hold up. If we were all more rational, we would see that the United States Public Health Service (USPHS) was actually responding to the gross disparities in health by allocating health care dollars to address a public health problem. In addition, White says that James Jones's highly respected, well-researched book about the TSS, "*Bad Blood*," is biased, sloppy, and laced with inaccuracies.

According to White, outrage over the study helps explain why the health of African Americans is worse than that of whites today. If African Americans got the real facts about the study, it would encourage us not to delay treatment, to participate in clinical trials, and to volunteer as organ donors. Discussing his version of the TSS would replace our outrage with reason. If we did this, White argues, we could be more active participants in effectively eliminating health disparities.

A University of Chicago anthropologist, Richard Shweder, maintained White's thesis in an Internet posting.[28] Shweder says he's tired of the accusations of racism regarding the TSS. He presents a "counternarrative" that flies in the face of the weight of existing analyses of the study. Shweder declares that the study was not racist, it did not harm the men, it did not make their lives worse, and they lived just as long as men who were treated for the disease. He goes on to say that rhetoric should be toned down because identity politics and political correctness have too heavily influenced conversation around the study.

Both White and Shweder have obscured the real issues. Their interpretation is a grave distortion of the facts, and their analyses are misleading. They are apologists for a shamefully racist experiment, and blatantly revisionist, as pointed out in numerous Internet responses by bioethicists. The TSS was built on lies and deception. The study remains a potent contributor to African American distrust of the health care system and is one reason why many African Americans refuse to participate in clinical trials.

Most chroniclers and experts on the study agree that little scientific merit came out of the experiment. However, debate around the ethical breaches of the study and the rights of research participants did lead to two important developments: the establishment of Institutional Review Boards (IRBs) to oversee human subjects research at hospitals, universities, and other research institutions, and the much-cited Belmont Report, a statement of basic principles to guide the ethical conduct of research with human subjects.

Story/Lie 4: *Statistical sleights of hand exaggerate and make things look worse than they are. For example, the number of smoking-related deaths in the United States has been grossly exaggerated.* This is the response of a Cato Institute Fellow and a retired employee of the National Bureau of Standards to a Centers for Disease Control and Prevention (CDC) report that stated that more than 400,000 people die per year from smoking-related deaths.[29]

The researchers, writing for the Cato Institute journal *Regulation*, blasted the CDC's smoking-death statistics in an article titled "Lies, Damned Lies, & 400,000 Smoking-Related Deaths."[30] They say the CDC's methodology was not reliable for several reasons: (1) the CDC study did not include representation from some populations; (2) the CDC did not correct for confounders such as obesity, high cholesterol, lack of exercise, and heart attacks that might have contributed to deaths among smokers; and (3) the 400,000 deaths were not an actual body count but a computer-generated estimate "based on assumptions biased by a political agenda of lies and loot."[31] They conclude that had CDC's researchers' work been less sloppy, the estimate of deaths due to smoking would have been reduced by one-third; that is, there are actually fewer than 270,000 smoking-related deaths per year.[32]

The director of the Office on Smoking and Health at the National Center for Chronic Disease Prevention and Health Promotion responded to the accusations in a letter to the editor of the *Philadelphia Daily News*.[33] The director's rejoinder: Statistical methods used by CDC are accurate and support the estimate of more than 400,000 deaths caused by smoking-related diseases. He further states that the Levy/Marimont article contained a number of errors that serve to minimize the harm of smoking, including life expectancy; for example, he reminds readers that 33 percent of nonsmokers live to age eighty-five, while only 12 percent of smokers live to that age.[34]

What has this to do with African Americans? Smoking is a major contributor to the three leading causes of death among African Americans: heart disease, cancer, and stroke. Lung cancer is the leading cause of cancer death in African Americans. Each year, approximately 45,000 African Americans die from smoking-related disease. African American men are at least 50 percent more likely to develop lung cancer and to die from it than white men. The incidence of cerebrovascular disease in African Americans is twice that in whites; African Americans are three to five times more likely to have a stroke than white Americans of the same age.[35]

The "statistical sleight of hand" argument has also been used by Alan Reynolds, a syndicated columnist at the Cato Institute, who argues that allegations that 44 million people are uninsured in this country are a statistical lie. He says that people typically have only short spells without health insurance and that many people who lack insurance choose not to have it.[36] Yet 11 percent of whites, 18.8 percent of African Americans, and 32.8 percent of Latinos were uninsured in 2003.[37]

As long as a large proportion of people—no matter their ethnicity—have difficulty getting preventive care and diagnostic and curative treatment, there will be health disparities between those who are insured and those who are not. To dismiss the deleterious effects of cigarette smoking and the lack of health insurance is to suggest that smoking is not as harmful as the CDC or the American Cancer Society would have the public believe, or that lack of health insurance in not a big national problem. This too flies in the face of thousands of epidemiological and clinical studies that show otherwise.

Story/Lie No. 5: *In some ways, the health of minorities is better than that of whites.* This is the conclusion of a Health and Human Services panel investigating health disparities. On December 23, 2003, the U.S. Department of Health and Human Services (HHS) released the National Healthcare Disparities Report (NHDR).[38] The report was supposed to be a comprehensive look at the scope and reasons for inequalities in health care. Amazingly, this final version of the report failed to mention several important observations that the IOM considered important, such as bias and scope of the disparities problem.[39]

Aware that a previous draft had supported the IOM findings, Representative Henry Waxman of California requested an investigation. The investigators found that an earlier July 2003 version did indeed agree with IOM findings. The July version was written by scientists at HHS.[40] Staff members at HHS subsequently rewrote the report, substantially changing the conclusion of the earlier version.

The new December version removed almost all occurrences of the word *disparity* and replaced it with the word *difference*. Thus there were no longer disparities in health care—only differences. This version eliminated references to the personal and societal costs of disparities. It omitted egregious examples of the disparities and instead highlighted milder examples. It eliminated the conclusion that the existence of health disparities is a national problem. It added that in some ways the health of minorities is better than that of the general population.[41] On February 11, 2004, in response to the Waxman investigation, Secretary Tommy Thompson admitted that his department had erred in rewriting the report and issued the original July 2003 version to the public in February 2004.

The second version of the report misled the public into thinking that the numerous reports on health disparities exaggerate the health status gap between whites and minorities. This public whitewashing of black health by government officials only does damage to the admirable work done by other government agencies. On the one hand, some government agencies/individuals try conscientiously to address a serious national problem. However, on the other hand, the attempts are diluted when other government entities distort the information to make things look better than they are. In addition, it reinforces the cynicism and mistrust of government, already rampant in communities of color.

Who Is Behind These Stories?
The Role of Corporate-Sponsored Think Tanks

These five stories came from conservative think tanks, individuals, and the government. The think tanks are noteworthy because they are a major source of newspaper and broadcast citations.[42] They reach huge audiences through media outlets they own or influence. They circulate their journals, magazines, and press releases to Congress, journalists, and congressional aides.

The conservative Cato Institute, American Enterprise Institute, and Heritage Foundation are the think tanks most frequently cited by the media.[43] The Cato Institute leads the push for privatizing government services. In 2001, the *Washington Post* noted that the Cato Institute spent about $3 million over a period of six years to advance the agenda for privatizing social services, including health care.[44] Among Cato's funders are Philip Morris, R. J. Reynolds, Chevron, Exxon, Shell, American Petroleum Institute, Eli Lilly, Merck, and Pfizer. The interests of the American Enterprise Institute include eliminating affirmative action. It has also been active in welfare reform. President George W. Bush has appointed more than a dozen people from the American Enterprise Institute to senior positions in his administration. People such as Charles Murray (of *The Bell Curve* infamy), ex-Enron chief Kenneth Lay, and Vice President Dick Cheney have been associated with the American Enterprise Institute. Corporate funders have included Shell, Corning Glass, and Alcoa.[45]

The Heritage Foundation has charted much of President Bush's domestic and foreign policy. It supports faith-based initiatives, a ban on abortion, and overturning affirmative action programs and is behind federal promarriage proposals that set aside $300 million for states to promote marriage—an initiative targeted at African Americans. The Heritage Foundation recognizes its great influence on legislators: "We generate solutions consistent with our beliefs and market them to the Congress, the Executive Branch, the news media and others."[46] Funders include General Motors, Ford Motor, Proctor and Gamble, Chase Manhattan Bank, Dow Chemical, the Readers' Digest Association, Mobil Oil, and GlaxoSmithKline Corporation.[47]

These think tanks have contributed to policies that negatively affect the health and well-being of African American and low-income communities. For example, the gutting of affirmative action, promoted by groups such as the Heritage Foundation, resulted in a decrease of minorities in medical school between 1995 and 2004. This is particularly harmful to black health because African American physicians are more likely to serve poor and minority communities than are white physicians. Conservative groups such as the American Enterprise Institute were instrumental in bringing about welfare reform, which left many African Americans and low-income parents and children without health care coverage.[48]

What Do These Stories Have in Common?

These five stories are not "mere" stories. And, indeed, it would be easy to find more such stories where individuals, think tanks, and the government concoct bogus narratives, for example, regarding the failures of affirmative action and Head Start, or why Social Security should be privatized, or why it is ethically justified for health providers to be involved in torture to retrieve information from detainees or prisoners of war. The previous stories serve a current political and economic worldview that favors the interests of multinational corporations—Big Tobacco, Pharma, and the petrochemical industries. Worldviews encompass beliefs about politics, economics, science, religion, culture, and ethics.

Assumptions derive from worldviews and result in public assertions that become part of the common discourse. The following section explores three assertions, or myths, inherent in the stories: (1) physician bias and racial stereotypes do not exist, (2) methodology in disparities research is seriously flawed and therefore useless, and (3) African Americans need to take responsibility for their poor health. Together, these three assertions weaken the struggle to end the disastrous condition of minority health.

Assertion 1: *Racial bias and stereotyping do not exist in the health care system.* We saw this assertion in Sally Satel's work;[49] we saw it in the Tuskegee discussion;[50] and we saw it in the recent HHS national report on disparities.[51]

Everybody agrees that African Americans are sicker and don't live as long as whites. There's no quarrel there. Several explanations have been proposed: We don't have sufficient access to the health care system; we don't have health insurance; we're too poor; our biology is different from that of whites, so medications don't work the same on us; communication with providers is of poor quality; we're uneducated or medically illiterate; and our attitude and behavior toward our health are irresponsible.

The IOM's study added another dimension: Physician bias contributes to racial health disparities. The IOM acknowledged that the bias was most likely unconscious. Physicians for Human Rights (an organization that promotes health internationally by protecting human rights, and a recipient of the 1997 Nobel Peace Prize) extended the IOM study. It compiled more than four hundred detailed annotations, analyzing and summarizing key research studies across a wide spectrum of disease categories and procedures. It too found that negative racial and ethnic stereotyping are persistent in health care structures.[52]

Do doctors think there is bias in health care? In a March 2002 Kaiser Foundation survey, over half of the doctors surveyed said that the health care system rarely treats people unfairly because of their race or ethnicity.[53] Thus their findings disagree with the IOM study. Of course, we all have biases that affect the decisions and judgments that we make about other people, and we are unaware of many of them. Does doctors' special clinical knowledge free them of unconscious bias? In one study, physicians tended to perceive African Americans as less intelligent, less likely to adhere to medical advice, and less rational than whites.[54] Does this indicate physician bias? Common sense suggests that most African Americans would think so.

What conditions are necessary for unconscious bias? Clinical uncertainty is one such condition, and it is normal: physicians can't know everything. Uncertainty about the risks and benefits of treatment can thus ethically justify different treatment. A second condition is physician discretion. Providers have a great deal of therapeutic discretion, and generally this is good and also ethically justified. But when clinical uncertainty and stereotypes meet head-on, they can influence how doctors use that discretion. For example, uncertainty and stereotyping could affect how providers communicate with blacks. Why spend valuable clinical time trying to communicate with people you don't believe can understand you? When clinical uncertainty leads to unequal and inferior care, racial biases and stereotyping may be a factor in clinical treatment.

Bias (unconscious or conscious) is not unique to medicine. It exists in housing, education, and job opportunities. Thus, to remedy bias in the health care system goes a long way, but it is not sufficient because of inequities in society at large.

Assertion 2: *Research methods are flawed.* The IOM study was portrayed as flawed in most of the stories because it was based on retrospective studies—analyses of peer-reviewed epidemiological and clinical research. This means that the IOM authors compiled and analyzed the results of other scientists. They did not go out and talk to actual people and ask such questions as "Was care offered?" "Did you accept or refuse?" Critics of the IOM report hypothesize that black patients often refuse care, which would explain why doctors give them less care. Rather than racial bias, then, it is patients' preferences that justify less or unequal treatment.[55] So the critics say that there is no evidence that doctors' prejudices lead to inferior care. We also saw that Fellows from the Cato Institute argued that faulty research methods exaggerated the number of smoking-related deaths. Yet it is well documented that smoking cigarettes causes chronic lung and heart disease and cancers of the lung, esophagus, larynx, mouth, and bladder, and smoking contributes to cancer of the pancreas, kidney, and cervix.[56]

Even so, how are we to respond to these accusations of flawed research? One response is that numerous research reports are based on retrospective studies. If retrospective studies are invalid for disparities research, shouldn't they be invalid for all studies? A second response is that most disparities research is published in prestigious and well-respected peer-reviewed journals such as the *Journal of the American Medical Association*, *The New England Journal of Medicine*, and the *American Journal of Public Health*. One purpose of peer review is to keep researchers honest. So most academics tend to trust the peer-review process, even though it may not be perfect.

Do the researchers at the Heritage Foundation, the Cato Institute, and the American Enterprise Institute go through peer review for their publications? Or are they really hired to sell policies to the president and to the media and to serve their funders? Murray, American Enterprise Institute Fellow—funded by the conservative Bradley Foundation—and Herrnstein bypassed peer review, and *The Bell Curve* became an influential bestseller, though subsequently denounced by the American Psychological Association. A *New England Journal of Medicine* reviewer lamented that the book had serious flaws and suggested that the book had not been peer reviewed.[57]

The avoidance of peer review by researchers such as Satel, Gough, and other detractors of disparities research make it more likely that it is their work that is methodologically flawed. Unproven accusations detract from the project of reducing health disparities and can be used to justify public and private inaction and inattention to the problem. In the short term, zealously accepting the mantra of flawed research could save the government and corporations hundreds of millions of dollars, but in the long term, millions of lives would be sacrificed and human potential unfilled.

Assertion 3: *African Americans must take more responsibility for their health.* All five stories allude to personal responsibility. This view lays the blame for poor health on the shoulders of minorities: the reason for increased cancers along Cancer Alley is due to smoking, not to toxic dumping; the environmental justice movement should not focus on cancers allegedly caused by pesticides; rather, it should focus its energy on encouraging African Americans to stop smoking (quite a worthy goal, especially when coupled with other initiatives). A few weeks after the IOM study came out, HHS secretary Tommy Thompson announced a national public relations campaign: "Take a Loved One to the Doctor Day." The purpose is to encourage minorities, particularly African Americans, to take charge of their own health by visiting a health professional. He targets African Americans because they are less likely to make routine visits to see a health professional. Secretary Thompson said that "Take a Loved One to the Doctor Day" would help eliminate health care disparities. The clear implication is that poor health is due to poor health habits, risky behavior, and the irresponsibility of not going for regular medical checkups.

Certainly, to a large extent, we are all responsible for our health—not only African Americans. All people should eat properly, exercise, get regular checkups, quit smoking, and so on. But laying the blame for poor health on the shoulders of racial and ethnic minority patients is an insufficient and disingenuous response to health disparities. It is a strategy of individualism that decontextualizes health disparities from the social system, thereby ignoring the social determinants of health: It discounts or minimizes the effect of not having health insurance, the shortages of providers in poor communities, the lack of transportation to health facilities, targeted cigarette advertising in communities of color, and the hazards of living in industrial wastelands or dangerous communities. By assigning blame to the individual, the strategy does not take into account inequities in the larger social system. It certainly ignores the role of unconscious bias in the health care system. As health inequalities are embedded in social inequalities, focus only at the individual level will not lead to wide-scale gains in reducing or eliminating health disparities.

Conclusion

I started with statements made by individual spokespeople. I moved on to the think tank organizations with which they are affiliated and then to a word about their corporate sponsors, which include tobacco, energy, and pharmaceutical companies, among many others. The individuals whom I mentioned are mouthpieces for the companies who fund them. They do not speak independently from their funding sources. For example, Robert Levy of the Cato Institute has published a number of articles in conservative journals, including the Cato journal *Regulation*, on the relative harmlessness of cigarette smoking. His articles do not disclose that Philip Morris and R. J. Reynolds are funders of the institute.[58] These think tank mouthpieces are influential liaisons between the corporations and the government and between corporations and the popular media.

Thus the stories told by scholars, researchers, and policy analysts are really coming from the corporations and are intentionally deceptive, that is, the stories are lies. As far back as 1944, for example, the American Cancer Society warned the public of the risks of smoking; in 1950, the *Journal of the American Medical Association* linked smoking to lung cancer; and the

1998 $200 billion tobacco settlement between states' attorneys general and the tobacco industry was an acknowledgment that companies had long been aware of the risks of smoking.[59] Similarly, Monsanto knew for forty years that its plant in Anniston, Alabama, was a toxic polluter but neglected to tell the mostly black community because, according to an internal memo, "We can't afford to lose one dollar of business."[60] Why are the corporations telling lies, making exaggerations, and vociferously denying the relation between their practices and citizens' health? Corporations and the government lie and deceive us not because they are inherently racist or malicious. They tell us these lies to serve their interests. The goal of corporations is to make money. While one of the roles of government is to secure economic health of the nation (by supporting business concerns), its support for business interests should not sacrifice the health and well-being of its citizens.

Let us briefly examine two examples where the misinformation campaigns and whitewashing can contribute to health disparities. Why do corporations lie about the relation between health and environmental pollutants? If, by lying, corporations can establish that environmental toxins are not serious health hazards, they are more likely to convince Congress and the public to deregulate petrochemical companies. Deregulation means less government oversight. Deregulation means more money for corporations: for example, price controls are lifted, industrial/chemical plants are located near poor and powerless communities, corporations can then more easily violate environmental laws, and they get to voluntarily monitor themselves. Poor people and communities of color live or work in these polluted areas; their health is disproportionately affected. And so the disparities continue.

Why would corporations lie about physician race bias? What's in it for them? In a privatized health care system, which is advocated by conservative think tanks, the goal is to make money. It has been shown over and over that fewer resources are used on blacks for a number of procedures, particularly in treating heart disease. Less resource use means more money for privatized health care systems. If health plans can establish that the lower resource use is not due to physician racial bias, but rather to "objective" clinical decisions, then the moral justification for providing fair treatment is weakened. It becomes clinical necessity—not physician bias and racism—that justifies different and less treatment.

To view health disparities purely as a medical problem is to overlook current political and economic trends and patterns. This country will not be able to achieve the humane goal of Healthy People 2010—eliminating health disparities—unless and until we understand and fight the problem at all fronts. This requires dealing not only with the clinical but also with the cultural, environmental, ethical, and—as I have argued here—the political and economic dimensions of health disparities.

Notes

1. U.S. Department of Health and Human Services, *Executive Summary: Report of the Secretary's Task Force on Black and Minority Health* (Washington, DC: U.S. Department of Health and Human Services, 1985).

2. *Trends in the Well-Being of America's Children and Youth*, 1997 ed., Office of the Assistant Secretary for Planning and Evaluation. U.S. Department of Health and Human Services (1997). Retrieved November 4, 2006, from http://aspe.hhs.gov/hsp/97trends/hc1-1a.htm

3. Donna L. Hoyert, Hsiang-Ching Kung, and Betty L. Smith, "Deaths: Preliminary Data for 2003," *National Vital Statistics Reports* 53, no. 15 (2005): 4.

4. M. F. MacDorman, J. A. Martin, and T. J. Mathews, "Explaining the 2001–02 Infant Mortality Increase: Data from the Linked Birth/Infant Death Data Set," in *National Vital Statistics Reports* (Bethesda, MD: National Center for Health Statistics, 2005).

5. National Center for Health Statistics, *Vital Statistics of the United States* (Rockville, MD: U.S. Department of Health, Education, and Welfare, 1970).

6. American Lung Association, "Trends in Asthma Morbidity, May 2005." Retrieved October 23, 2006, from www.lungusa.org/site/pp.asp?c=dvLUK9O0E&b=33309; National Center for Health Statistics, "Asthma Prevalence."

7. John C. Nelson, *Testimony to the Sullivan Commission on Diversity in the Healthcare Workforce* (Chicago: AMA, 2003).

8. *Journal of Blacks in Higher Education*, "A Journal of Blacks in Higher Education Check-up on Blacks in U.S. Medical Schools" (2005). Retrieved November 4, 2006, from www.jbhe.com/features/47_medicalschools.html

9. Institute of Medicine, "Unequal Treatment: Confronting Racial and Ethnic Disparities in Health Care" (Washington, DC: National Academies Press, 2002).

10. Sally Satel, "Racist Doctors? Don't Believe the Media Hype," *Wall Street Journal*, April 4, 2002.

11. Sally Satel and Jonathon Klick, *The Health Disparities Myth: Diagnosing the Treatment Gap* (Washington, DC: American Enterprise Institute, 2006); Sally Satel, "Health and Medical Care," in *Beyond the Color Line: New Perspectives on Race and Ethnicity in America*, ed. Abigail Thernstrom and Stephen Thernstrom (Stanford, CA: Hoover Press, 2002), 127.

12. Sally Satel, *PC, MD: How Political Correctness Is Corrupting Medicine* (New York: Basic Books, 2002).

13. Sally Satel and Christine Stolba, "Who Needs Medical Ethics?" *Commentary* 111, no. 2 (2001): 37–40.

14. Satel, "Racist Doctors?"

15. Christopher Foreman, "Environmental Justice and Risk Assessment," *Human and Ecological Risk Assessment* 6, no. 4 (2000): 549–54.

16. Michael Gough, "Did You Hear? Good News from Cancer Alley" (1997). Retrieved October 24, 2006, from www.junkscience.com/news/canceralley.html

17. Robert Bullard, *Dumping in Dixie: Race, Class, and Environmental Quality* (Boulder, CO: Westview Press, 1990); IOM, *Toward Environmental Justice: Research, Education and Health Policy Needs* (Washington, DC: National Academy Press, 1999), 65.

18. Barbara Koeppel, "Cancer Alley, Louisiana," *The Nation*, November 8, 1999, vol. 269, pp. 16–24; John McQuaid, "'Cancer Alley': Myth or Fact?" *The Times-Picayune*, May 23, 2000, p. A9.

19. Foreman, "Environmental Justice."

20. Gough, "Did You Hear?"

21. IOM, *Toward Environmental Justice.*

22. Gough, "Did You Hear?"

23. Koeppel, "Cancer Alley"; McQuaid, "Myth or Fact?"

24. United Health Foundation, "America's Health: State Health Rankings—2004 Edition" (November 8, 2004). Retrieved October 23, 2006, from www.united healthfoundation.org/shr2004/Findings.html

25. National Cancer Institute, "State Cancer Profiles: Death Rates" (2005). Retrieved October 23, 2006, from http://statecancerprofiles.cancer.gov/deathrates/ deathrates.html

26. R. M. White, "Unraveling the Tuskegee Study of Untreated Syphilis," *Archives of Internal Medicine* 160, no. 5 (2000): 585–98.

27. Ibid.

28. Richard Shweder, "Tuskegee Re-Examined" (2004). Retrieved October 25, 2006, from www.spiked-online.com/articles/0000000CA34A.htm

29. CDC, "Annual Smoking: Attributable Mortality, Years of Potential Life Lost, and Economic Costs—United States, 1995–1999," *Morbidity and Mortality Weekly Report* 51, no. 300 (2002).

30. Robert A. Levy and Rosalind B. Marimont, "Lies, Damned Lies, & 400,000 Smoking-Related Deaths," *Regulation* 21, no. 4 (1998): 24–29.

31. Rosalind Marimont, "Casualties of the War on Smoking—Truth, Freedom, Fairness, and Children Forces International" (1997). Retrieved October 24, 2006, from www.forces.org/articles/files/roz-03.htm

32. Levy and Marimont, "Lies."
33. Michael P. Eriksen, "The Official Answer of the CDC to the Levy/Marimont Letter" (1999). Retrieved October 23, 2006, from www.data-yard.net/10/cdca.html
34. Ibid.
35. CDC, "African Americans and Tobacco Information and Prevention Sources (TIPS)" (1998). Retrieved October 24, 2006, from www.cdc.gov/tobacco/sgr/sgr_1998/sgr-min-fs-afr.html
36. Alan Reynolds, "Politicized 'Facts'" (2003). Retrieved October 24, 2006, from www.catoinstitute.com/research/articles/reynolds-031005.html
37. Carmen DeNavas-Walt, Bernadette D. Proctor, and Robert J. Mills, "U.S. Census Bureau, Current Population Reports, P60-226," *Income, Poverty, and Health Insurance Coverage in the United States, 2003* (Washington, DC: U.S. Government Printing Office, 2004). Retrieved November 6, 2006, from www.census.gov/hhes/www/hlthins/hlthin03/hlthtables03.html
38. Agency for Healthcare Research and Quality, "National Health Disparities Report" (2003). Retrieved October 28, 2006, from www.house.gov/reform/min/politicsandscience
39. IOM, *Unequal Treatment.*
40. Agency for Healthcare Research and Quality, "National Healthcare Disparities Report" (July 2003). Retrieved November 3, 2006, from http://qualitytools.ahrq.gov/disparitiesreport/archive/2003/download/download_report.aspx
41. Gregg M. Bloche, "Health Care Disparities: Science, Politics, and Race," *New England Journal of Medicine* 350, no. 15 (2004): 1568–70.
42. World Information Organization, "Report: Fact and Opinion Construction (Think Tanks) Table: Media References to Major U.S. Think Tanks World Information Organization" (2005). Retrieved November 2, 2006, from http://world-information.org/wio/infostructure/100437611704/100438658270?opmode=contents
43. Ibid.
44. Glenn Kessler, "Paving the Way for Privatizing Social Security," *Washington Post,* June 26, 2001, p. A1.
45. People for the American Way, "Right Wing Watch People for the American Way" (2002). Retrieved November 3, 2006, from www.pfaw.org/pfaw/general/default.aspx?oid=4456
46. Heritage Foundation, "About Heritage" (June 19, 2005). Retrieved November 4, 2006, from www.heritage.org/About/aboutHeritage.cfm
47. Ibid.
48. Jane L. Holl, Kristen Shook Slack, and Amy Bush Stevens, "Welfare Reform and Health Insurance: Consequences for Parents," *American Public Health Association* 95, no. 2 (2005): 279–85.

49. Satel, *Political Correctness,* and "Racist Doctors?"; Sally Satel and Jonathan Klick, "Too Quick to Diagnose Bias," *Perspectives in Biology and Medicine,* suppl. no. 48, vol. 1, no. 1 (2005): S15–S25; Satel and Stolba, "Who Needs Medical Ethics?"

50. Shweder, "Tuskegee Re-Examined"; White, "Unraveling."

51. Agency for Healthcare Research and Quality, "National Health Disparities Report, 2003."

52. Physicians for Human Rights, "The Right to Equal Treatment: An Annotated Bibliography of Studies on Racial and Ethnic Disparities in Health Care, Their Causes, and Related Issues." Report by the Panel on Racial and Ethnic Disparities in Medical Care. Retrieved November 3, 2006, from www.phrusa.org/research/domestic/race/race_report/bibliography.html

53. Kaiser Family Foundation, "National Survey of Physicians: Part I. Doctors on Disparities in Medical Care." The Kaiser Family Foundation survey (2002), p. 22.

54. M. Van Ryn and J. Burke, "The Effect of Patient Race and Socio-Economic Status on Physicians' Perceptions of Patients," *Social Science and Medicine* 50 (2000): 813–28.

55. Satel, *Political Correctness,* and "Racist Doctors?"

56. J. L. Fellows et al., "Annual Smoking-Attributable Mortality, Years of Potential Life Lost, and Economic Costs: United States, 1995–1999," *MMWR* 51, no. 14 (2002): 300–303.

57. Daniel M. Fox, "Review of *PC, M.D.: How Political Correctness Is Corrupting Medicine,*" *New England Journal of Medicine* 344, no. 6 (2001): 462.

58. People for the American Way, "Right Wing Watch."

59. Tobacco Free, "Highlights of Tobacco History" (2005). Retrieved November 4, 2006, from www.tobaccofreeqc.org/youth/history_of_tobacco.shtml

60. Michael Grunwald, "Monsanto Hid Decades of Pollution: PCBS Drenched Ala. Town. But No One Was Ever Told," *Washington Post,* January 1, 2002, p. A01.

CHAPTER 4

Race, Equity, Health Policy, and the African American Community

Patricia A. King

Herein lie buried many things which if read with patience may show the strange meaning of being black here at the dawning of the Twentieth Century. This meaning is not without interest to you . . . for the problem of the Twentieth Century is the problem of the color line . . . the relation of the darker to the lighter races of men in Asia and Africa, in America and the islands of the sea.

W. E. B. Du Bois, *The Health and Physique of the Negro American*

In order to get beyond racism we must first take account of race. There is no other way. And in order to treat some persons equally, we must treat them differently.

Justice Harry A. Blackmun

In 1903, W. E. B. Du Bois, the acclaimed African American scholar, writer, and activist, wrote that the color line would be the problem of the twentieth century. In retrospect, it appears that he was prophetic, but his timeline was too optimistic. One hundred years later, at the beginning of the twenty-first century, the color line remains a problem for American society.

To be sure, important strides have been made toward achieving equality for African Americans, especially in the last half of the twentieth century. In the landmark 1954 decision of *Brown v. Board of Education of Topeka*,[1] the

Supreme Court unanimously held segregation in public schools unconstitutional. During the 1960s, federal laws, notably the Civil Rights Act of 1964, were enacted to end Jim Crow laws and other legal barriers maintaining segregation and to achieve racial equality in American society.[2]

Nonetheless, at the beginning of the twenty-first century, disparities between blacks and whites persist[3] in every sector of American life, including income, educational achievement,[4] and housing.[5] Racial inequality continues because there is continuing discrimination by whites against blacks[6] and because of the cumulative effects of America's legacy of slavery and segregation. In this century, it is still important to attend to the problem of how people are treated because of their race and to employ race-based strategies as necessary to accomplish the goal of achieving equality.[7] Justice Blackmun's insight is as perceptive today as it was in 1978.

Persistent social and economic inequalities in the society provide the context for large disparities in health outcomes and in health care that exist between blacks and whites in the United States.[8] According to Geiger, "At no time in the history of the United States has the health status of minority populations . . . equaled or even approximated that of white Americans."[9] Despite gains in disease prevention, minorities have not enjoyed the same gains as white Americans in terms of health. Racial and ethnic minorities continue to bear a disproportionate share of the burden of illness and death. For example, approximately 40 percent of African American men and women have some form of heart disease, compared with 30 percent of white men and 24 percent of white women. African Americans are also 29 percent more likely to die from cardiovascular disease than are whites. Similarly, African Americans are 23 percent more likely to die from cancer than are whites. The prostate cancer incidence rate among African American men is 60 percent higher than the rate in white men, and the prostate cancer death rate is more than twice as high among African Americans as any other racial or ethnic group.[10] Although the rate of newly diagnosed cases of breast cancer is about 13 percent lower than in white women, African American women have higher mortality rates than any other racial or ethnic group.[11]

The reasons for differences in health status among population groups are complex. Social, physical, and economic environments are viewed as major contributors to these disparities. The impact of these factors in turn is linked to the norms and values of the broader society that shape the way critical resources and opportunities are distributed.[12]

Racial and ethnic disparities in health care exist as well.[13] In 1999 Congress asked the Institute of Medicine (IOM) to "assess the extent of racial and ethnic differences in healthcare that are not otherwise attributable to known factors such as access to care" and "to evaluate potential sources of racial and ethnic disparities in healthcare, including the role of bias, discrimination, and stereotyping at the individual, institutional, and health system levels."[14] The IOM report issued in response to this congressional charge made a key finding. It states, "Bias, stereotyping, prejudice, and clinical uncertainty on the part of healthcare providers may contribute to racial and ethnic disparities in healthcare."[15] While addressing racial and ethnic disparities in health care will bring progress, these efforts alone will be insufficient. It will also be necessary to broadly address social and economic inequality in the society, for example, in housing, education, and employment, before substantial gains in eliminating inequalities in health status can be made.

Americans, however, are not of one mind about the norms and values that should be invoked in determining whether or how society should respond to racial disparities in health status and health care. "What divides Americans," according to Michael Brown and others, "is profound disagreement over the legacy of the civil rights movement. At the core of our national debate are very different opinions about the meaning of race in contemporary America and the prospects for racial equality in the future."[16] Does race still matter? Has equality been achieved? What are the causes of racial disparities in health and other sectors of our national life? The debate is ongoing, in part because these questions are placeholders for larger ones: How should African Americans fit into society? How and to what extent should we correct for historic injustice? Are blacks the same or different from whites or other minorities? What role does health play in achieving social justice?

These questions touch upon cherished and deeply held values of fairness and equality in society. At the core of the country's understanding of itself is that all persons in the same or similar position should be treated similarly. The benefits and burdens that flow from public policy and expenditure must be distributed irrespective of race. This view of the meaning of equality is expressed in the Supreme Court's opinion in *Brown v. Board of Education of Topeka*, where the Court states, "Separate educational facilities are inherently unequal."[17] The color of one's skin is irrelevant, or in the frequently quoted words of Justice Harlan in *Plessy v. Ferguson*, "Our Constitution is color-blind."[18] Even though this ideal has not been the reality for African Americans in the health care system or in other domains of American life, the aspiration is of continuing importance. On this view, the gap in health outcomes and in health services between blacks and whites should illicit no special governmental response, because it would be unfair, and possibly in some circumstances illegal, to use racial classification in an effort to advance the interests of African Americans.

This color-blind or race-neutral approach has been fiercely debated in the decades since *Brown* was decided. The *Brown* opinion itself is susceptible to multiple interpretations. For example, it can be argued that the Court was focused not merely on dismantling segregation but rather on what segregation signified. Not only were the races separated, but segregation also implied the superiority of whites and the inferiority of blacks. Racial subordination and not mere racial separation was the core issue.[19] Judge Robert Carter, who, along with Thurgood Marshall, argued the *Brown* case before the Supreme Court, made this point when he wrote many years later, "It was not until Brown I was decided that blacks were able to understand that the fundamental vice was not legally enforced racial segregation itself; that this was a mere by-product, a symptom of the greater and more pernicious disease—white supremacy."[20] The implication in Judge Carter's statement is that, while segregation could be ended with a legal requirement of color blindness, the disease of white supremacy could not be so easily eradicated.

Using a color-blind or race-neutral approach is unfair because racism persists, and this approach makes it unlikely that blacks will ever be able to close the social and economic gap created by centuries of slavery, segregation, and subordination. President Lyndon Johnson, in a famous speech at Howard University on June 4, 1965, said it best: "You do not take a person who, for years has been hobbled by chains, liberate him, bring him up to the starting line of a race, and then say, 'you are free to compete with all the others,' and still justly believe that you have been completely fair."[21] In short, a color-blind approach preserves the status quo and the inequities that persist between blacks and whites.

A view of equality that incorporates race-conscious policies is necessary to ameliorate or eradicate continuing vestiges of white supremacy, including the elimination of racial disparities in health and the health system. "There is widespread basis for agreement," in the words of Powers and Faden, "that inequalities in health outcomes that track racial and ethnic lines, especially when racial and ethnic lines track other indices of social disadvantage, are ethically problematic."[22] Moreover, they urge "a special moral sensitivity to the constellation of race, ethnicity, and social disadvantage when we have ample reason to believe that . . . racial differences have made a dramatic contribution to the disproportionate burdens that are an artefact of the social structure."[23] Clearly, the debate about the meaning of equality is relevant to whether and how this society confronts racial disparities in health outcomes and health care.

In American medicine and research, race has been used both to advance and to adversely affect the health interests of African Americans. Historically, the health needs of African Americans were ignored except to the extent that they were relevant to the needs of whites. Because blacks were not only powerless but also considered inferior to whites, their helplessness was exploited in educational, medical, and experimental projects to further the health interests of whites. Significantly, however, since the 1990s, a few race-conscious policy initiatives have been employed in the health system in efforts to fairly distribute health benefits. Changes in kidney transplantation allocation policies is one well-known example.[24] The kidney allocation policy example, because it grapples with human leukocyte antigens (HLA) matching, suggests that race-conscious policies may be needed in future circumstances where it is important to capture genetic variation across human populations.[25]

As a practical matter, both race-conscious and race-neutral policies pose significant challenges. While race-neutral policies seem to be consistent with the goal of attaining equality, they do not adequately address lingering effects of burdens imposed on African Americans during slavery and segregation. In contrast, race-conscious policies, where they are used, have the potential for undermining the core vision of equality for all. Thus they should be limited in duration and employed no more broadly than the purpose of their use demands. Indeed, the country for much of its history used race-conscious policies to deny blacks opportunities available to whites, and this history should make us wary about using them. From the perspective of African Americans, particularly worrisome is the possibility that, by emphasizing racial disparities in health and promoting efforts to eliminate them, race-conscious policies may perpetuate misconceived notions of race and increase burdens for African Americans by fostering stigmatization and stereotyping. Indeed, the IOM report, which takes the position that data should be collected with racial identifiers, also finds that stereotyping is a major contributor to unequal treatment in health care. These concerns are heightened when the goal of eliminating racial disparities in health intersects with genetic research. Conversely, what is different today is that race-conscious policies are being advocated with the intent of furthering, not hindering, equality. Moreover, as worrisome as fear of perpetuating race, stigmatization, and stereotyping is, this fear must be balanced against the harm that flows from ignoring the reality that racism persists in the culture.

In this chapter I recount how the debate about the meaning of equality is emerging in medicine and research. My personal sympathies lie with those who favor race-conscious approaches. Surely, more than forty years are needed to surmount the obstacles posed by four hundred years of slavery, segregation, and subordination. I do not mean, however, simply to reprise the race-neutral/race-conscious debate. Rather, I wish to make the point that the debate is oversimplified as applied to racial disparities in health services and health outcomes. The debate in its simplified form omits nuance and complexity, which is the place where the possibility for convergence and dialogue about rectifying racial disparities lies. I argue that achieving racial equality in the health system, as in other sectors of society, requires a mix of race-neutral and race-conscious policies and strategies in order to achieve equality. What is critical is that, in both its conception and implementation, the strategy employed should be consistent with achieving the end that is sought.[26] That end is a society that has rid itself of racial hierarchy. In medicine, which employs genetic knowledge in research and clinical practice, there may be circumstances where the use of race-conscious policies is problematic, because such policies may impede rather than further equality for blacks. By contrast, using racial identifiers to collect and organize data might be useful in uncovering structural features of the health delivery system that impede the delivery of quality health care to African Americans. In the effort to eliminate racial disparities in health, it is important to critically examine health system policies and their implementation to determine whether the use of race contributes to or detracts from the elimination of the continuing legacy of subordination and racial hierarchy. This chapter concludes by raising important questions about using race in scientific and medical research in order to illustrate the complex issues raised in efforts to reduce racial disparities in health status and in health care.

Americans Divided about Race and Ethnic Disparities in Health

The debate about the meaning of equality is being played out in the health arena as in other domains of American life. Why do African Americans lag so far behind whites in health status, and what is the role of government and health institutions in confronting these disparities?

Racial disparities in health status and health outcomes have a long history that can be traced to slavery and before. Dr. W. E. B. Du Bois documented in detail the existence of these disparities in his book *The Health and Physique of the Negro American*, in 1906. Although the gap between blacks and whites in health has long existed, governmental efforts to address these problems are of recent vintage. Discrimination in health care institutions and programs receiving federal assistance was formally ended in 1964. Yet it was not until 1984, with the establishment of the Task Force on Black and Minority Health to examine health issues of blacks and other minorities, that federal efforts to confront racial disparities in health really began. The task force's report, issued in 1985, marks a shift in the federal government's concerns about black health status.[27] The report called attention to significant gaps that existed in scientific knowledge on the health status of African Americans and other minorities and noted the need for greater inclusion of racial and ethnic minorities in research. Beginning in the 1990s minority health issues have received increased attention. In 1990 the National Institutes of Health (NIH) Office of Research on Minority Health was created. In 1993 Congress passed a statute that requires NIH to ensure that women and minorities are included in the study populations of all NIH-funded research. In 1998 President Clinton announced the goal of eliminating racial and ethnic disparities by the year 2010, and in the following year, Congress passed legislation requiring the Agency for Healthcare Research and Quality (AHRQ), a part of the Department of Health and Human Services, to report annually to Congress on racial, ethnic, socioeconomic, and geographic disparities in health care. In the first years of the twenty-first century, several reports confirmed the existence of racial disparities in health care and offered strategies for their elimination. For example, the IOM report on racial disparities in health care found that racial disparities in health care exist and are unacceptable. They also concluded that the disparities were extensive and made detailed findings, conclusions, and recommendations about what was required to address them adequately.[28]

Although federal efforts are ongoing, Americans disagree profoundly about the nature and significance of racial inequities in health care, particularly in their understanding of the social changes from the 1960s to the present. They disagree about the explanations for the existence of disparities and consequently disagree about the appropriate actions for their correction.

Americans diverge, in a very fundamental way, in their interpretation of the significance of historical practices for present-day realities. For race-conscious policy advocates, knowledge and appreciation for the past raise fundamental issues of justice and equality, offer important lessons, and provide strong reasons for affirmative or compensatory interventions in the present. There is a concern about the legacy of past practices and persistent adverse effects of unconscious bias and, in particular, the potential of facially neutral practices to disproportionately impact African Americans.

The past serves as a reminder of the harm that can flow from race-conscious practices and policies. As one author puts it, "Health is arguably the site where the legacy of racial discrimination is borne most harshly upon the body."[29] Policies and practices historically relied on inadequate scientific and biological explanations for health disparities and susceptibility to disease. For many, eugenics and social Darwinism are not merely distant memories, but rather frequently resemble modern beliefs and practices that promote stigmatization and negative stereotypes as well as reinforce differences in ways that retard rather than promote attention to the problem of disparities in health. Although racial differences in health outcomes are complex with multiple interacting causes, historically and today, there is a tendency to overemphasize genetic explanations and the contributions that genetic research can make to alleviate disparities in health.[30]

Some advocates of race-conscious policies prefer to focus on the future. While there is knowledge and appreciation of the past, there is also concern that too much emphasis on the past is counterproductive, divisive, and encourages finger-pointing. Race-conscious interventions are justified not to rectify past injustice but as a means of bringing about a more just society in the future. For example, those who believe that a healthier workforce is required for the nation's economic future might be willing to collect and utilize racialized data if collection of such data would further this goal.

Many other Americans reject entirely the argument that the shadow of past racial practices looms over contemporary life. They believe that social problems should be viewed in their current dimensions only and that the past should be put behind us. They are not persuaded that society should give special attention to racial disparities in health today, in part because they urge that discrimination and inequality have been significantly diminished.

An example of this approach involved efforts to amend the California constitution through the initiative process. The Racial Privacy Initiative (Proposition 54) was the brainchild of Ward Connelly, a person best known for proposing and getting enacted California Proposition 209, which banned the use of affirmative action in California state universities. Proposition 54 would have prohibited the state from collecting and using data about a person's race, ethnicity, color, or national origin in the operation of public education, public contracting, or public employment.[31] Proponents argued that Proposition 54 would be a first step toward a color-blind society. Because the U.S. Constitution prohibits discrimination on the basis of race, there is no need to classify people. Indeed, they argued, classification by race fosters division and brings undue attention to differences between individuals and groups rather than emphasizing common interests. Finally, proponents would add that, because information derived from the Genome Project shows that there is no biological basis for race, there is no reason to engage in practices that seemingly affirm nineteenth-century notions of race in the sense that all members of a race have characteristics that differ from other races.

Proposition 54 did contain an exemption that allowed classification of medical research subjects and patients, but critics argued that the exemption was imprecise, ambiguous, and only allowed physicians to keep racial data on their patients. Consequently, Proposition 54 would hinder the ability to address disparities by race and ethnicity in public health.

What the Polls Tell Us

These divisions among Americans emerge with clarity in polling data. In general, whites are more optimistic than minorities about whether significant progress has been made. A *Washington Post*/Kaiser Family Foundation/Harvard University survey in 2001 indicated that 51 percent of Americans polled (only 23 percent of African Americans polled) believe that African Americans have "about the same opportunities in life as whites have," and slightly fewer (49 percent) said the same of Hispanics.[32] When polled about access to health care, 50 percent of whites said African Americans were "just about as well off as the average white person," and 42 percent said the same of Hispanics. By contrast only 26 percent of African Americans and 33 percent of Hispanics agreed that they were just as well off as the average white person. In another national poll conducted by Lake Snell Perry Associates in 2003 for Harvard University, 52 percent of whites, but only 22 percent of African Americans, believe that whites and minorities receive equal quality of care.[33]

Similarly, the majority of doctors believe that the health care system "rarely" or "never" treats people unfairly based on racial or ethnic background

(55 percent, rarely; 14 percent, never).[34] Twenty-nine percent of doctors say the health care system "very often" or "somewhat often" treats people unfairly based on their race or ethnicity, but minority doctors disagree. Seventy-seven percent of black physicians and 52 percent of Latino physicians say this unfair treatment occurs "very often" or "somewhat often." In general, physicians are less likely to think that the health care system treats people unfairly based on what their race or ethnic background is (29 percent of physicians as opposed to 47 percent of the public surveyed, an 18 percent-point gap).

The data tend to show that whites believe that equality has been achieved or nearly achieved in health care, while blacks have strongly divergent views. Whites see "differences," and blacks see racism and continuing discrimination. What explains this divergence in views about the urgency with which these disparities must be attacked?

As the polls indicate, many Americans believe that there is no serious problem. Racial disparities are not a significant matter. Blacks have made significant progress and should therefore elicit no special concern. A somewhat recent controversy underscores the policy implications of these divisions and demonstrates that this view is often at work among policymakers. In July 2003, AHRQ submitted a draft of the congressionally mandated annual report on health disparities for departmental approval. In December 2003 the report that was released was notably different from the draft. Differences between the two drafts were detailed in a staff report, prepared for Representative Henry Waxman and seven other democratic representatives. The key findings were that most uses of the word *disparity* were deleted, the final report no longer viewed disparities as "national problems," and finally, that key examples of health care disparities were omitted. The controversy ended when Secretary Tommy G. Thompson announced on February 10, 2004, that the original draft would be released without changes.[35] The major differences between the two versions of the report lie in the use of the term *disparity* and the implications that should be drawn from the data. Indeed, the December version states, "Where we find variation among populations, this variation will simply be described as a 'difference.' By allowing the data to speak for themselves, there is no implication that these differences resulted in adverse health outcomes or imply prejudice in any way." The December version finds that priority populations do as well or better than the general population in some aspects of health care.[36] Obviously, if there is no significant problem, there is little or no reason for governmental intervention to reduce inequalities.

Does Inequality Imply Injustice?

Many agree that significant disparities in health between whites and blacks exist, but disagree about whether the existence of these disparities implies continuing inequality or injustice that should trigger governmental or other forms of social intervention. Some point to the progress that has been made since the 1960s to emphasize that racial inequality in health should not be of current concern. They argue that the Constitution and other laws that prohibit intentional and purposeful discriminatory acts are sufficient to regulate the behavior of individuals in the health system who might still seek to inflict harm on African Americans. The polls discussed earlier show, for example, that the attitudes and beliefs of whites have changed over time. Thus it can be argued that whites no longer erect barriers to access and equal treatment. Rather, differentials in health status and health care can be explained by the lack of personal responsibility among blacks or in attitudes, practices, and beliefs inimical to health that are deeply embedded in black culture. For example, psychiatrist Sally Satel focuses on the patient and emphasizes patient needs or patient attitudes and beliefs to explain disparities in health. She argues, "The nature of their belief in their personal susceptibility to disease, the seriousness with which they perceive disease, their confidence that treatment will work—and even that the medical system is benign—are all relevant."[37] In addition, she contends "uneven access to medical services, disparate knowledge of good health practices and personal attitudes . . . underlie the vast majority of differences in health outcomes."[38]

Although there has indeed been progress in achieving equality since the 1960s, the claim should not be overstated. Those who claim that racial injustice and inequality persist point to the inadequate enforcement of the law prohibiting discrimination in the health care system. The United States Congress formally ended unequal treatment of blacks and whites in the health care system with the passage of Title VI of the Civil Rights Act of 1964. This provision prohibited discrimination based on race, color, or national origin in any program or activity receiving federal financial assistance. Although Title VI does not explicitly contain the word *health*, the expanding federal role in health care, along with judicial and legislative clarifications of Title VI's scope, has ensured that this provision reaches most health care activities in the United States.[39] Title VI applies to both intentional discrimination—acting with intent or purpose to discriminate—and the application of policies and practices neutral on their face, but that have the effect of discriminating on the basis of race—disparate impact or effects test.[40]

Although the impact of Title VI has been substantial, many argue that its promise as a tool to end racial inequality in the health care system remains unfulfilled. On the one hand, despite enormous resistance, enforcement of the federal law opened access by black patients to formerly segregated hospitals and desegregated hospital wards. On the other hand, federal regulations issued pursuant to Title VI do not offer adequate compliance instructions to health care institutions.[41] Since the Supreme Court's 2001 holding in *Alexander v. Sandoval* that Title VI did not create a private right of action absent of discriminatory intent, thus ending the use of disparate impact or effects test for private causes of action, the responsibility for compliance monitoring and enforcement of Title VI rests with the federal government. Many argue that federal enforcement has been inadequate. For example, the United States Civil Rights Commission has issued a very critical report of the enforcement of Title VI by the Office of Civil Rights in the Department of Health and Human Services.[42]

Moreover, race-conscious proponents argue that a requirement for intentional and purposeful acts ignores much of what we know about human behavior. What the passage of Title VI did accomplish was the establishment of a mechanism to rectify intentional, random, and individualized acts. The context in which African Americans lived, worked, and sought access to health care, however, remained the same. Desegregating hospitals and hospital wards did not mean that African Americans would be able to easily access those institutions or health care generally, or if access were achieved, that African Americans would be treated with dignity. Hospital doors and wards were open to all, but institutional policies and practices remained unchanged.

Those who argue for color-blind policies today fail to appreciate that those current inequalities and practices in society, including in the health care system, are linked to earlier times in which the cultural meaning of institutional practices and processes were manifest. The effects of unintentional choices of individuals and the institutional policies and practices that support those choices still matter. Americans share a history and culture in which racism has been a powerful force. Consequently, individuals may not perceive how their conduct has been affected by cultural practices, beliefs, and attitudes. They may not be aware of their unconscious motivation. As the IOM report "Unequal Treatment" recognized, adverse consequences for patients might flow from unconscious behavior. The IOM defined discrimination to be "differences in care that result from biases, prejudices, stereotyping, and uncertainty in clinical communication and decision-making."[43]

To be sure, there is a significant role for individual responsibility in our health system. The view that patients' attitudes are responsible for disparities in health care and health outcomes is overly simple, however. Is it realistic to be able to separate individual responsibility from social responsibility? For example, it is widely accepted that African Americans distrust the health system and that this distrust has roots in the Tuskegee Syphilis Study and other abuses in research and health care that date back to slavery. One could argue that individual and collective mistrust of the health system by African Americans, to the extent that it results in inadequate diagnosis and treatment, is their own responsibility. This is to ignore however, that "what will count as reasonable will depend upon people's past experiences, the likelihood and extent of the possible harm, and the resources that are available to cope with any bad eventualities."[44] The Tuskegee Syphilis Study is a case of clear violation of the rights of African American research subjects. When confronted with other public health communicable disease crises, it is not unexpected that African Americans might believe history is repeating itself.[45]

Further, given the difficulty of disentangling responsibility for individual health as between the individual and society, we should err on the side of those who historically have been and today are socially disadvantaged and carry a disproportionate burden. This is especially the case when the issue at stake—health status and health outcome—is considered one of the basic human goods.

Class Inequality Rather Than Race Inequality?

Among those who agree that current data indicate that racial disparities in health between blacks and whites exist and should be eliminated with governmental assistance are those who urge that the real culprit is class, not race, inequalities. They urge that because many Americans who are in low-income categories are also racial and ethnic minorities, the greatest benefits from intervention are likely to flow from tackling classist rather than racial inequalities.[46] In other words, they advocate a shift in focus away from racial disparities to a focus on improving the overall health of the public. To be sure, there are significant methodological and data collection problems in compiling data by socioeconomic levels in a nation that has historically ignored class divisions, but it is believed that, with time and will, these issues can be overcome.[47] Because a class-oriented approach would help both poor whites and poor blacks, many believe that moving in this direction is fairer and would enjoy wider and deeper public support.

The danger in this class versus race discussion is that it ignores strong reasons to have data arrayed along both race and class lines. Black poverty is not white poverty. For example, infant mortality rates are higher among African Americans than among whites, even when comparing women of similar socioeconomic condition as measured by years of education completed.[48] Many of the causes of infant mortality among both the poor and African Americans, as well as many of the interventions required to alleviate high infant mortality rates, are likely to be the same. But there are differences between the two groups, and these differences are racial in nature to the extent that they reflect the African American experience in America.

Hurricane Katrina very dramatically unmasked the nature and complexity of poverty, race, class, and inequality in America. After the storm at least two things were clear. First, poverty and economic inequality remain major social problems for the country. Whether a person was able to evacuate New Orleans before the storm arrived depended in part on whether he or she had access to transportation. More than half of poor households in New Orleans did not have a vehicle in 2000.[49] Second, in America, race still matters. Katrina burdened some victims more than others. It is commonly accepted that the burden was heaviest on African Americans who lived in the lowest-lying areas. One in three African American households and nearly three in five poor African American households were without a vehicle in 2000. African American households were twice as likely as white households to be without an automobile, thus making it difficult to leave the city before the storm arrived.[50] Even President George W. Bush, while calling attention to the poverty in the Gulf region, acknowledged indirectly that race was an issue, when he said that "poverty has roots in a history of racial discrimination which cut off generations from the opportunity of America."[51] Race and class are inextricably linked but they are not the same.

The essence of the race-conscious argument is that inequality is cumulative and persistent with deeply embedded roots in the past. While intentional discrimination is prohibited, systemic practices and processes remain virtually untouched, and affirmative race-conscious efforts are required. Race-neutral strategies are ineffective in tackling these sorts of practices, and it is necessary to take some risks in order to make progress. Both race-neutral and race-conscious strategies are means to an end that the vast majority of Americans affirm. Because race-conscious approaches potentially undermine this goal, they must be used with care to address problems and practices that race-neutral approaches cannot effectively address.

Race consciousness may not always be necessary or wise. A problem in one area of the health system may justify race-conscious approaches that should not be utilized in other domains. For example, race-conscious approaches might be needed to increase the number of African Americans in health professions.[52] These approaches might not justify, however, using race categories in federally funded clinical research. Policies or practices should be assessed individually within a framework that seeks to identify the potential benefits and risks of using race-conscious policies, to evaluate methods for reducing risks, and to consider possible alternatives to race-conscious policies. A brief consideration of this framework in the context of the use of racial variables in biomedical research illustrates the complexity of such assessments.

Using Race as a Variable in Medical Research

W. E. B. Du Bois, in his account of disparities between blacks and whites in *The Health and Physique of the Negro American*, posed the critical question that always arises when attention is drawn to differences between blacks and whites. He wrote: "The undeniable fact is, . . . that in certain diseases the Negroes have a much higher rate than the whites, and especially in consumption, pneumonia and infantile diseases. The question is: Is this racial?"[53]

Are health status differences between blacks and whites innate, and thus indicative of inferiority, or can these disparities be explained by social and economic factors, including discrimination, bias, and stigmatization in the health care system itself? Du Bois clearly believed that social and economic conditions were primarily responsible for the disparities he documented. His efforts showed the importance of being able to document the health status of blacks. He was well aware, however, that data about racial disparities could be used against black interests to demonstrate the inherent inferiority of blacks.

The authors of a more recent article published in 1992 pose a related question. "Is racial research in medicine racist?"[54] Osborne and Feit focus on whether medical research using race as a variable is conducted in a manner that fosters genetic rather than economic, social, or political explanations for differences between blacks and whites. Socioeconomic status is highly cor-related with racial and ethnic categories. Frequently race is used as a proxy for socioeconomic status or environmental impact on health. While such re-search may bring important health information to African Americans who are of low socioeconomic status, using race as a proxy may also send the message that race, rather than economic status, is the contributor to disease or poor health. Osborne and Feit do not suggest that the use of racial vari-ables should be eliminated entirely but rather urge that continued use poses serious obstacles for science. For example, there is no definition of race that is scientifically acceptable. Consequently, to categorize research subjects by race and ethnicity creates a perception of mutual exclusiveness that is not warranted. They argue that researchers must "explain the reason(s) for se-lecting (or excluding) variables."[55] Scientists must also "define terms clearly, [and] state the hypothesis on which the studies are based."[56]

Osborne and Feit were prescient. Today there are even more urgent rea-sons to address the questions they raised. There has been a huge increase in the comparative research studies they discuss. In addition, a growing num-ber of research studies are genetic studies of complex traits.[57]

In 1993 Congress passed the National Institutes of Health Revitalization Act.[58] This statute requires that NIH ensure that women and minorities are included in the study populations of all NIH-funded research.[59] Inclusion of African Americans in clinical research has resulted in increased reporting of research results by racial categories. The legislation responded to several con-cerns relevant to women and racial minorities; there was worry that the health issues pertinent to women and minorities were being ignored. These "inclusion requirements" were instituted for laudable reasons, and they re-flect important values in American medicine and research.

Those who support the use of racial categories in research despite recog-nition of its ambiguity and lack of precision argue that it is necessary to identify and monitor health issues for blacks. They argue that there is value in using race as a proxy for a vast array of social, economic, and environ-mental factors that are not measured directly but are disproportionately dis-tributed across socially constructed racial and ethnic groups. In other words, race identifiers are required in order to help eliminate racial and ethnic dis-parities in health care and delivery.

Information from the Human Genome Project has generated a vast amount of information about human variation that has further complicated discussions about using race as a variable. On the one hand, this information supports the conclusion that there is no biological basis for race in the sense that human variation is coextensive with socially constructed categories of race and ethnicity. For the most part, all humans are alike, and variation is overwhelmingly at the individual rather than at the population level. In other words, there is nothing that all whites possess and all blacks do not. Variation is continuous across all socially constructed racial and ethnic groups. That is the good news.

On the other hand, medicine is appropriately interested in exploring human differences at the molecular level, if understanding differences might lead to more effective therapies for all. Differences in the frequency of alleles that might play a role in susceptibility to disease or response to therapeutic interventions may correlate with socially constructed racial and ethnic groups. The debate, then, is not over whether human populations differ genetically. They do. The debate is over the scientific, clinical, and social significance of labeling biological difference as race.

The question then arises whether research designed to detect medically important differences among humans should utilize race variables as proxies for geographic ancestry. And, if such use can be justified in at least some circumstances, how can the reification of race in its historical sense be avoided? In the social sphere, race has attributes that despite attempts cannot be separated from its meaning. Socially constructed race has been used not only to create a classification scheme for populations but also to explain inherent attributes of the social order, according to which some groups dominate and are superior to others. In sum, how should variation in human populations be characterized? Should race be used in its social sense, or should, for example, genetic markers be used to "cluster" humans into populations? Although there are ongoing efforts to show that such "clustering" through genetic markers is feasible theoretically and practically, science is not there yet. In the meantime, what can be done to advance knowledge, including information relevant to relieving the burden of illness and disease for blacks, while at the same time mitigating the burdens for blacks that will inevitably flow from equating race with human difference?

There are clearly uses of racialized data that potentially benefit African Americans. These benefits may go beyond just the identification of gaps between blacks and whites.[60] For example, an article and editorial in the *New England Journal of Medicine* gives credence to the view that use of race in studies of health outcomes can be beneficial to African Americans. The researchers started with the premise that black patients typically receive a lower quality of care than do white patients. They hypothesized that perhaps black patients were receiving care from a subgroup of physicians that were less qualified or less able to obtain services for patients than those who treat white patients. They found that black patients and white patients were largely being cared for by different physicians. Further, they determined that these two groups of physicians differed in rates of board certification and in physicians' reported ease of access to services for their patients. Finally, they suggest that detected differences flowed from the characteristics of physicians who practice where black and white patients receive care. Thus differences were the result of the distribution of physicians and not patients' preferences. The large majority of black patients' visits were with white physicians. The editorial accompanying the study stated that the report indicates that "structural features of the [health] delivery system . . . also contribute to racial disparities in the quality of care."[61] The study points to a complex delivery system and interaction between quality of care and other indicators of broad societal discrimination, thus offering some evidence in support of structural explanations for racial inequality in health care delivery. Such work is important because it points to structural forces, not individual preferences, as the explanation for inequities, thus providing support for a societal obligation to remedy the problem of racial disparities in health.[62]

Using race variables in other contexts is more complicated. Some of the most convincing evidence of racial disparities in health care comes from studies of cardiovascular care. While, realistically speaking, the prospect of tailoring treatments by individuals is probably not going to be possible for quite a while, if ever, individual members of racial and ethnic groups may potentially benefit from emerging information about correlation between race and susceptibility to disease or response to therapeutic interventions. Drug research is especially promising. The African American Heart Failure Trial (A-HeFT), sponsored by NitroMed, Inc., is a clinical study that established the efficacy of BiDil among black patients with advanced heart failure.[63] This trial is the first to enroll exclusively self-identified African American patients. Preliminary trials had demonstrated no statistically significant effect in white patients but suggested that African American patients could have a different and more positive reaction to treatment.[64] In June 2005, the Food and Drug Administration (FDA) approved BiDil based on A-HeFT's results.[65]

As the first drug to be approved because of efficacy based on race, BiDil has been the subject of much debate and controversy. Critics question the validity of the drug approval, which was based on a clinical trial involving African Americans only and, therefore, did not prove ineffectiveness in other population groups.[66] NitroMed admits that the biological basis for BiDil's clinical benefits are unknown, so thus far, there is no biological support for race being the reason why BiDil works in African Americans. The result, critics agree, is a reification of race and biological difference.[67]

BiDil supporters counter that "race may be the coarsest of discriminators,"[68] but the results of A-HeFT reflect that it can still be a valid proxy for a collection of genetic traits that, in the absence of better evidence, speak of a relationship between genes, heart disease, and responsiveness to therapy.[69] BiDil's manufacturer and researchers are attempting to understand the mechanism that makes BiDil effective—a mechanism that is present in some but not all African Americans and individuals of other population groups. Discovery of that mechanism will likely mean moving beyond racial classifications and lead to targeting potential BiDil beneficiaries based on nonracial means—possibly genetic testing. Meanwhile, supporters highlight that the result of using race in this case benefits African Americans, a population that has suffered a disproportionately high burden of heart disease compared to whites, and that denying the unique benefit of BiDil to African Americans would be a mistake.

Even if African Americans disproportionately benefit, the question remains whether other drugs are likely to be developed for the purpose of offering new therapeutic options for blacks. There is evidence to suggest that BiDil was developed for economic and commercial purposes independent of any desire to help African Americans.[70] Moreover, at the time of this writing, BiDil has been on the market for a little more than a year, and sales have been disappointing. BiDil is reaching only 1 percent of African Americans with heart disease.[71] Poor utilization of the drug is due to a number of factors, including NitroMed's pricing of the drug, resistance by insurers to cover the drug, and a change in federal policy affecting former recipients of Medicaid who were also covered by Medicare Part D.[72] As a consequence of poor sales, NitroMed has had to reduce its sales staff. The company's financial woes may discourage companies from pursuing race-specific therapies in the future. The BiDil episode to date illustrates well that effectively reducing disparities between blacks and whites requires more than merely developing new therapeutics.

Many agree that the use of racial categories in research is not desirable, but may be needed as an interim measure, and that in the future variations may be detected without the need to use racial and ethnic categories. They argue that the use of racial categories is required to provide information on which personalized medicine can be developed, thus eliminating the future need for the categories altogether.[73] In the meantime, however, personalized medicine is many decades away. Moreover, as the development of BiDil suggests, there is also the potential for targeting groups, not individuals, before individualized therapeutic interventions are scientifically and economically feasible. In the interim, research policies and practices should be designed to reduce the likelihood that information about human variation will be used to elevate some population groups over others. Research practices should seek to overturn and eliminate racial inequalities in medicine, not reify race. The significant contemporary issue is how to ensure that using race in research contributes to the elimination of, rather than reinforcing, racial inequality in the health system. If race categories are to be used, they must be employed with care to minimize the potential for harm. How might race variables be employed with greater care in biomedical research? Many issues need to be examined before that question can be answered. The critical ones will be raised here.

At the outset, investigators and reviewing authorities should ask whether race as a variable should be used at all. Are there appropriate and inappropriate uses of race as a variable in research? If so, can they be described?[74] Are there feasible alternatives that are more accurate and precise? Where race is being used, how is it being defined? For example, is it being used to point to disadvantage and discrimination? Or is it being used to link a phenotypic characteristic with a specific socially constructed group?

Under NIH guidelines, study sections and Institutional Review Boards are charged with the responsibility for reviewing the research applications involving inclusion policies. Both those who advocate the use of racial categories and those who argue for discontinuation of their use appreciate that harm resulting from bias, discrimination, or stigmatization of subjects might occur. They differ in beliefs about the value of the scientific knowledge that might be gained, and the degree of risk and magnitude of harm that might result. Do those who conduct, review, and publish research employing racial variables need a fuller understanding of the nature of the harm that results from stigma and the role it plays in stereotype formation? How are people determined to be in one racial group as opposed to another? Current requirements allow subjects to self-identify. What do we know about what self-identification measures? Are subjects reflecting biological, socioeconomic, or cultural constitutive aspects of themselves? Moreover, self-identification may be problematic in face of increasing heterogeneity. Growing intermarriage and immigration creates heterogeneity within broad categories. For example, Cuban Americans might be considered black or white after arrival in the United States depending on their skin color. Can we be confident that subjects, rather than third parties, place themselves in these categories? Do subjects have the opportunity to self-identify, or are they placed in categories by those who enroll them? If this happens frequently, how are such classifications made? By skin color? By some other method based on law or ancestry or country of origin? Can we improve our utilization of self-identification by making more precise social classifications?

Further, how should research results be reported? Can standards and best practices to guide investigators and journals be developed? As two authors point out, "For discussion of disparities to be meaningful and precise, equal attention should be given to the way in which race and ethnicity are conceptualized and described and the rationale for reporting racial/ethnic differences."[75] The use of racial categories creates problems not only for science and medicine to the extent that they are not precise measures but also for the broader society. Presentation of research results as neutrally and precisely as possible, particularly with respect to racial implications, benefits all.

Conclusion

When W. E. B. Du Bois wrote that the color line was the problem of the twentieth century, he was too optimistic. Achieving equality for African Americans in this country will be a problem for the twenty-first century as well. In this century, Americans must grapple with whether race-conscious polices can be employed to eliminate or reduce racial disparities in health and, if utilized, how they should be conceptualized and implemented. The manner in which research studies are designed and carried out has enormous significance for how the resulting knowledge will be used. Efforts to alleviate these disparities, without at the same time causing a backlash, will be challenging. Nowhere is the challenge greater than at the intersection of emerging genetics research and racial disparities in health.[76]

Notes

1. 347 U.S. 483 (1954).
2. Public Law 88-352, 78 Stat. 241 (1964; Codified as amended at 2000, 42 U.S.C. [2002]).
3. Neil J. Smelser, William Julius Wilson, and Faith Mitchell, "National Research Council," in *America Becoming: Racial Trends and Their Consequences* (Washington, DC: National Academy Press, 2001).
4. James Smith, *Race and Ethnicity in the Labor Market: Trends over the Short and Long Term.* Vol. 2, *America Becoming: Racial Trends and Their Consequences* (Washington, DC: National Academy Press, 2001).
5. Douglas Massey and Nancy Denton, "American Apartheid: Segregation and the Making of the Underclass," in *American Apartheid* (Cambridge, MA: Harvard University Press, 1993).
6. Civil rights law has traditionally focused on employment, housing, recipients of public funding, and public accommodations. Discrimination, however, may occur in retail markets such as in car negotiations where blacks and whites are treated differently, or in "unconventional" markets where policies have disparate impact on blacks, as in access to kidneys. See Ian Ayres, *Pervasive Prejudice? Unconventional Evidence of Race and Gender Discrimination* (Chicago: University of Chicago Press, 2001).
7. This chapter focuses on African Americans or blacks even where I use the term "minorities." Although the United States is increasingly a multicultural society, and a focus on differences between blacks and whites fails to capture demographic complexity, I concentrate on African Americans because the black experience in America is distinctly different from that of immigrants or refugees. This is due to the extended period of slavery, the persistent discrimination over centuries, and the use of skin color as a metaphor for dehumanization of black persons.
8. Raymond S. Kington and Herbert W. Nickens, *Racial and Ethnic Differences in Health: Recent Trends, Current Patterns, Future Directions.* Vol. 1, *America Becoming: Racial Trends and Their Consequences* (Washington, DC: National Academy Press, 2001).
9. H. Jack Geiger, "Racial and Ethnic Disparities in Diagnosis and Treatment: A Review of the Evidence and a Consideration of Causes," in *Unequal Treatment: Confronting Racial and Ethnic Disparities in Health Care*, ed. Brian D. Smedley, Adrienne Y. Stith, and Alan Nelson (Washington, DC: National Academy Press, 2003), 417–54, 417.
10. Department of Health and Human Services, "Minority Health Disparities at a Glance," ed. The Initiative to Eliminate Racial and Ethnic Disparities in Health, U.S. Department of Health and Human Services, 2004.

11. Ibid.
12. Gary King, "Institutional Racism and the Medical/Health Complex: A Conceptual Analysis," *Ethnicity and Disease* 6 (Winter/Spring 1996): 30–46.
13. American Medical Association, Council on Ethical and Judicial Affairs, "Black-White Disparities in Health Care," *Journal of the American Medical Association* 263 (1990): 2344–46.
14. Brian D. Smedley, Adrienne Y. Stith, and Alan Nelson, eds., *Unequal Treatment: Confronting Racial and Ethnic Disparities in Health Care* (Washington, DC: National Academy Press, 2002), 30.
15. Ibid., at 12.
16. Michael K. Brown et al., *White-Washing Race: The Myth of a Color-Blind Society* (Berkeley: University of California Press, 2003), 1.
17. 347 U.S. 483, 492.
18. 163 U.S. 537, 558 (1896).
19. Kathleen Sullivan, "What Happened to 'Brown'?" *The New York Review of Books* 51, no. 14 (2004): 47.
20. Robert Carter, "A Reassessment of *Brown v. Board*," in *Shades of Brown: New Perspectives on School Desegregation* (New York: Teacher's College, Columbia University, 1980), 23.
21. Lyndon B. Johnson, Commencement Address at Howard University: "To Fulfill These Rights" (Washington, DC: U.S. Government Printing Office, 1965). Retrieved December 12, 2006, from www.lbjlib.utexas.edu/johnson/archives.hom/speeches.hom/650604.asp
22. Madison Powers and Ruth Faden, "Racial and Ethnic Disparities in Health Care: An Ethical Analysis of When and How They Matter," in *Unequal Treatment: Confronting Racial and Ethnic Disparities in Health Care*, ed. Smedley, Stith, and Nelson (Washington, DC: National Academy Press, 2003), 22–38, 729.
23. Ibid., at 734–35.
24. Ayres, *Pervasive Prejudice*, 165–232.
25. Ruth R. Faden et al., "Public Stem Cell Banks: Considerations of Justice in Stem Cell Research and Therapy," *Hastings Center Report* 33 (2003): 13–27.
26. Amy Gutmann, "Responding to Racial Injustice," in *Color Conscious: The Political Morality of Race* (Princeton, NJ: Princeton University Press, 1996), 106–78.
27. Todd Savitt, "Minorities as Research Subjects in the Encyclopedia of Bioethics," in *Encyclopedia of Bioethics*, vol. 3 (New York: Simon and Schuster Macmillan, 1995), 1776–80.
28. Smedley, Stith, and Nelson, *Unequal Treatment*.
29. Lynn M. Sanders, "All Things Equal?" *Du Bois Review* 1, no. 1 (2004): 195, 201, 197.
30. Pamela Sankar et al. "Genetic Research and Health Disparities," *Journal of the American Medical Association* 291, no. 24 (2004): 2985–89.

31. Retrieved from www.adversity.net/rpi/rpi_mainframe.htm

32. Kaiser Family Foundation, *Washington Post*, and Harvard University, "Toplines—Race and Ethnicity in 2001: Attitudes, Perceptions, and Experiences" (report of Kaiser Family Foundation, *Washington Post*, Harvard University, 2001), 1–57.

33. Lake, Snell, Perry, & Associates, "Americans Speak out on Disparities in Health Care—Results from a National Poll" (Poll conducted by Lake, Snell, Perry & Associates, 2003), 1–7.

34. Kaiser Family Foundation, "National Survey of Physicians. Part I, Doctors on Disparities in Medical Care" (The Kaiser Family Foundation survey, 2002), 1–22.

35. Robert Steinbrook, "Disparities in Health Care: From Politics to Policy," *The New England Journal of Medicine* 350, no. 15 (2004): 1486–88.

36. United States House of Representatives Committee on Government Reform Minority, "A Case Study in Politics and Science: Changes to the National Healthcare Disparities Report" (2004). Retrieved December 12, 2006, from www .democrats.reform.house.gov/features/politics_and_science/pdfs/pdf_politics_ and_science_disparities_rep.pdf

37. Sally Satel, *PC, MD: How Political Correctness Is Corrupting Medicine* (Washington, DC: AEI Press, 2000), 166.

38. Ibid., 232.

39. P. Preston Reynolds, "Hospitals and Civil Rights, 1945–1963: The Case of *Simkins v. Moses H. Cone Memorial Hospital*," *Annals of Internal Medicine* 126, no. 11 (1997): 898–906; Lynn Marie Pohl, "Long Waits, Small Spaces, and Compassionate Care: Memories of Race and Medicine in a Mid-Twentieth-Century Southern Community," *Bulletin of the History of Medicine* 74, no. 1 (2000): 107–37.

40. Thomas E. Perez, "The Civil Rights Dimension of Racial and Ethnic Disparities in Health Status," in *Unequal Treatment: Confronting Racial and Ethnic Disparities in Health Care*, ed. Smedley, Stith, and Nelson (Washington, DC: National Academy Press, 2003), 626–63.

41. Ibid., 640.

42. United States Commission on Civil Rights, "Health Care Challenge: Acknowledging Disparity, Confronting Discrimination and Ensuring Equality," in *United States Commission on Civil Rights, Health Care Challenge* (Washington, DC: U.S. Government Printing Office, 1999).

43. Smedley, Stith, and Nelson, *Unequal Treatment*, 4.

44. Howard McGary, "Distrust, Social Justice, and Health Care," *The Mount Sinai Journal of Medicine* 66, no. 4 (1999): 236–40, 238.

45. Stephen Thomas and Sandra Quinn, "The Tuskegee Syphilis Study, 1932 to 1972: Implications for HIV Education and AIDS Risk Education Programs

in the Black Community," *American Journal of Public Health* 81, no. 11 (1991): 1498–1505.

46. Stephen Isaacs and Steven Schroeder, "Class: The Ignored Determinant of the Nation's Health," *The New England Journal of Medicine* 351, no. 11 (2004): 1137–42.

47. Ibid.; N. Krieger, D. R. Williams, and N. E. Moss, "Measuring Social Class in U.S. Public Health Research," *Annual Review of Public Health* 18 (1997): 341–78.

48. Kaiser Family Foundation, "Key Facts: Race, Ethnicity & Medical Care" (2003). Retrieved December 12, 2006, from www.kff.org/minorityhealth/6069-index.cfm

49. Arloc Sherman and Isaac Shapiro, "Essential Facts about the Victims of Hurricane Katrina" (2005). Retrieved December 12, 2006, from www.cbpp.org/9-19-05pov.htm

50. Ibid.

51. George W. Bush, Address to the Nation on Hurricane Katrina (2005). Retrieved December 12, 2006, from www.whitehouse.gov/news/releases/2005/09/20050915-8.html

52. Sullivan Commission, "Missing Persons: Minorities in the Health Professions—A Report of the Sullivan Commission on Diversity in the Healthcare Workforce" (report of the Sullivan Commission, 2004), 1–201.

53. W. E. B. Du Bois, *The Health and Physique of the Negro American* (Atlanta, GA: Atlantic University Press, 1906).

54. Newton G. Osborne and Marvin D. Feit, "The Use of Race in Medical Research," *Journal of the American Medical Association* 267, no. 2 (1992): 275–79, 275.

55. Ibid., 276.

56. Ibid.

57. Alexandra E. Shields et al. "The Use of Race Variables in Genetic Studies of Complex Traits and the Goal of Reducing Health Disparities: A Transdisciplinary Perspective," *American Psychologist* 60, no. 1 (2005): 77–103.

58. National Revitalization Act, Public Law 88-352, 78 Stat. 241 (1964; Codified as amended at 2000, 42 U.S.C. [2002]).

59. The FDA has issued a draft, "Guidance for Industry: Collection of Race and Ethnicity Data in Clinical Trials," which indicates that the FDA will adopt the Office of Management and Budget's racial and ethnic group categories for use in drug development and research. At the time of this writing, the FDA has not finalized its proposal. The document is available at www.fda.gov/cber/gdlns/raceth clin.htm

60. Peter B. Bach et al. "Primary Care Physicians Who Treat Blacks and Whites," *The New England Journal of Medicine* 351, no. 6 (2004): 575–84.

61. Arnold M. Epstein, "Health Care in America: Still Too Separate, Not Yet Equal," *The New England Journal of Medicine* 351, no. 6 (2004): 603–5, 604.

62. Elizabeth H. Bradley et al. "Racial and Ethnic Differences in Time to Acute Reperfusion Therapy for Patients Hospitalized with Myocardial Infarction," *Journal of the American Medical Association* 292, no. 13 (2004): 1563–73.

63. Anne Taylor et al. "Combination of Isosorbide Dinitrate and Hydralazine in Blacks with Heart Failure," *The New England Journal of Medicine* 351, no. 20 (2004): 2049–57.

64. Jonathan Kahn, "How a Drug Becomes 'Ethnic': Law, Commerce, and the Production of Racial Categories in Medicine," *Yale Journal of Health Policy, Law and Ethics* 4, no. 1 (2004): 1–33.

65. Department of Health and Human Services (2005). Retrieved December 12, 2006, from www.fda.gov/cder/foi/appletter/2005/020727ltr.pdf

66. M. Gregge Bloche, "Race-Based Therapeutics," *The New England Journal of Medicine* 351, no. 20 (2004): 2035–37.

67. Jonathan Kahn and Pamela Sankar, "Being Specific about Race-Specific Medicine" (2006). Retrieved December 12, 2006, from http://content.healthaffairs.org/cgi/content/full/hlthaff.w5.455/DC1

68. Gary Puckrein, "BiDil: From Another Vantage Point" (2006). Retrieved December 12, 2006, from http://content.healthaffairs.org/cgi/content/full/hlthaff.25.w368v1/DC1

69. Rick J. Carlson, "The Case of BiDil: A Policy Commentary on Race and Genetics" (2005). Retrieved December 12, 2006, from http://content.healthaffairs.org/cgi/content/full/hlthaff.w5.464/DC1

70. Kahn, "How a Drug Becomes 'Ethnic,'" 1–33.

71. Sylvia Pagan Westphal, "Heart Medication for Blacks Faces Uphill Battle" (2006). Retrieved December 12, 2006, from www.post-gazette.com/pg/06289/730462-114.stm

72. Ibid.

73. Elizabeth G. Phimister, "Medicine and the Racial Divide," *The New England Journal of Medicine* 348, no. 12 (2003): 1081–82; Mark A. Rothstein and Phyllis Griffin Epps, "Ethical and Legal Implications of Pharmacogenomics," *Nature Reviews Genetics* 2 (2001): 228–31.

74. R. Dawn Comstock, Edward M. Castillo, and Suzanne P. Lindsay, "Four-Year Review of the Use of Race and Ethnicity in Epidemiologic and Public Health Research," *American Journal of Epidemiology* 159 (2004): 611–19.

75. Judith B. Kaplan and Trude Bennett, "Use of Race and Ethnicity in Biomedical Publication," *Journal of the American Medical Association* 289, no. 20 (2003): 2709–16.

76. Pamela Sankar et al., "Genetic Research and Health Disparities," *Journal of the American Medical Association* 291, no. 24 (2004): 2985–89; Shields et al., "Use of Race Variables," 77–103.

CHAPTER 5

Religion and Ethical Decision Making in the African American Community: Bioterrorism and the Black Postal Workers

Cheryl J. Sanders

IN THE weeks following the September 11, 2001, attack on the World Trade Center and the Pentagon, some letters containing deadly anthrax spores were mailed to two senators on Capitol Hill, leading to the first cases of bioterrorism-related anthrax in the United States. As they were processed and delivered through the mail system, the contaminated letters caused twenty-two cases of anthrax, and among them five fatalities. Nine postal employees associated with the postal facilities that processed the letters in Trenton, New Jersey, and in Washington, D.C., contracted anthrax. Two employees from the Brentwood facility in Washington, D.C., died.

The mailing of letters laced with anthrax exposed a troubling dimension of our nation's public health and emergency response systems, namely, that the health and well-being of postal workers did not warrant the same immediate attention and intense measures as were given to the senators, congresspersons, and their staffs on Capitol Hill. It was obvious that the letters mailed to Senator Tom Daschle of South Dakota and Senator Patrick Leahy of Vermont had to have been handled by the U.S. Postal Service. Yet the testing of postal facilities and administration of antibiotics to postal workers did not occur until after two postal workers, Joseph Curseen Jr. and Thomas Morris Jr., had died from inhalation anthrax (despite their own efforts to seek emergency medical treatment in a timely fashion).

Largely because they exempt themselves from the civil rights regulations and affirmative action rules they have imposed on others, our nation's legislators and their assistants maintain an overwhelmingly white presence on Capitol Hill. By contrast, the vast majority of postal workers in Washington, D.C., are black, as may be expected in a city with a majority black population. Thoughtful observers within and outside the U.S. Postal Service quickly pointed to racial discrimination as a factor in determining who got attention, testing, and treatment in this tragic sequence of events.

When antibiotics and vaccines were finally offered to the postal workers who had possibly been exposed to anthrax, most of them refused or discontinued treatment. Their reasons included fear of unpleasant side effects (such as nausea, vomiting, diarrhea, abdominal pain, dizziness, and erectile dysfunction) and fear of being used as human guinea pigs by the Centers for Disease Control (CDC):

> "It's now time to trust in God," said Rudolph Trotter, 53, of Upper Marlboro, a Brentwood carrier who quit after three days on Cipro. "I figure He has a better answer than CDC has. He's kept me." Celia Chambers, 44, of Clinton, said she never started the drug regimen. "Believe me, I'm okay," she said. "I trust in God—that's the bottom line." Betty Primes, a mail handler and 23-year postal worker, said she and others are frustrated by the CDC's equivocal answers. "It's more like they're guessing—they don't know exactly, either," she said. "When I wanted to know the long-term side effects of using these drugs, they couldn't answer. . . . I thought they were using us as guinea pigs, like we're being experimented on."[1]

Similar suspicions were expressed by postal workers with respect to the government's offer of a free anthrax vaccine: "Echoing the comments of numerous postal workers interviewed in recent days, Brentwood worker Delancy Praylow, Jr. said he was suspicious of the vaccine, and would not take it. He has not taken any antibiotics, either. 'I trust in God only,' he said."[2]

In March 2002 it was reported that only 152 of more than 5,100 exposed postal workers accepted the federal government's offer of anthrax vaccine, which is to say that an overwhelming majority of 97 percent refused treatment.[3]

The postal workers' refusal to protect themselves against deadly inhalation anthrax using remedies offered by the government is a clear manifestation of their mistrust of both the medicine and the government. Their decision to countenance the threat of death without trusting medicine is fueled by well-founded suspicions of racial bias in the administration of public health decisions. But awareness of racism seems not to be the only factor here. While voicing their skepticism regarding the antibiotics and vaccines, many asserted their determination to "trust in God" for healing and protection.

The anthrax attack presents an interesting case study of the role of religion in responses to bioterrorism. The impact of African American religion and health practices can be readily discerned in the resistant attitudes and behavior of the black postal workers in this situation. In addition, there are historical precedents underlying their concern for unequal treatment and fear of being used by the government as "guinea pigs." In this chapter I highlight two features of the peculiar responses of the black postal workers to the clear danger of anthrax inhalation: on the one hand, a folk religion that engenders faith in divine healing and protection, and on the other, an awareness of the history of racial discrimination in American medical practice, which brings a persistent threat to bear upon the health and well-being of African Americans.

"I Trust in God": Folk Healing and Medical Science in Conflict

Although a careful assessment of the African origins of African American folk health practices lies well beyond the scope of this chapter, it is important to approach the study of African American religious belief and practice with some sense of the long legacy of African traditional beliefs. In African religions and culture, "health is not a personal matter but is related to the well-being of the whole community. The right relationship with God and with the whole community gives peace. Real health is to be found in a balanced relationship between one's body, soul and spirit, between those around one, such as a harmonious relationship with the congregation and with the metaphysical forces of which God is the highest. Healing thus concerns the whole person in his individuality and communality."[4]

Writing with respect to the African American context, historian Albert J. Raboteau has described the important interactions of sacred medicines and spirit possession in African traditional approaches to healing, noting that "for the African traditional healer . . . medicine was not enough to effect a cure without the presence of ritual that made medicine effective. Ritual was necessary because illness and cure involved the spiritual, not just the material."[5]

The African tradition holds that "prayer and song worked as medicine alongside the teas and poultices."[6] Beverly Robinson highlights the positive contributions African healing traditions and practices brought to bear on American life:

America's early pioneering health practices were greatly influenced by the enslaved Africans' concern for health, well-being, and preventive medicine. In fact, this concern is a result of the institutionalized system of slavery, which mandated that enslaved Africans rely on a holistic form of survival as a consequence of their economic, political, and social status.

Africans in America, like European colonial settlers, possessed their own materia medica, which proved to be of value not only for their own health but for the health of all of early America. One instance is the "buying of the smallpox—a method of inoculation designed to prevent the onset of this dread disease by the use of a serum from human patients having the infection in a mild form." In Igboland of West Africa this method was used to control local outbreaks of smallpox. Knowledge of birth by cesarean section and snake-bite cures are among the other medical contributions Africans brought to America.[7]

Notwithstanding occasions when healing practices and information were shared across boundaries of race, culture, and class, for the most part African American folk healers were resisted and ridiculed by representatives of the dominant culture. In her insightful study of slave women's healing practices, Sharla Fett notes that while slave women derived authority and leadership in their own communities as healers, wielding their knowledge of signs and of medicinal herbs and roots as an arsenal against the dangers of ill health and slaveholder violence, not surprisingly they "found their judgment and methods as healers frequently questioned by slaveholders, physicians, and overseers."[8] Moreover, African American slave women healers were empowered to claim spiritual insight, divine calling, and communally derived authority, clearly undermining slaveholder views of them as subservient assistants.[9]

Throughout the African American sojourn from slavery to freedom, the interaction of ancient notions of sacred medicine and spirit possession lived on in the worship of black "shouting" churches. On the basis of this historical and ecclesiological premise, Raboteau posits his understanding of African American healing practices firmly within the Holiness-Pentecostal tradition, or the sanctified church. He cites reports of healing among black Pentecostals from the September 1906 inaugural issue of *The Apostolic Faith*, the newspaper of the Azusa Street revival: "Many have laid aside their glasses and had their eye sight perfectly restored. The deaf had the hearing restored. . . . A man was healed of asthma of twenty years standing. Many have been healed of heart trouble. . . . A little girl who walked with crutches and had tuberculosis of the bones, as the doctors declared, was healed and dropped her crutches and began to skip about the yard."[10]

The special significance of the Holiness-Pentecostal emphasis emerges in view of two considerations: ritual and piety. The healing rituals of the tradition evoke biblical and cultural images of spirit possession: "Preachers and evangelists transmitted the healing power of the Spirit by the laying on of hands. Healing in the Holiness-Pentecostal tradition came also by anointing with oil, by using blessed water, and by applying prayer cloths to the sick body."[11] In his overview of the Pentecostal tradition published in the anthology *Caring and Curing: Health and Medicine in the Western Religious Traditions*, Grant Wacker insists that the majority of Pentecostal leaders "urged total avoidance of professional help, and many displayed overt hostility toward the medical and especially pharmaceutical professions."[12]

Loudell Snow has done several studies of the contemporary folk health beliefs and practices of the African American poor, and her informants are largely identified with the Holiness-Pentecostal tradition. Her research, published in medical journals, gives attention to the healing as a spiritual gift. She acknowledges the relatively low ranking of the medical practitioner in this scheme:

> The ability to heal is seen as being a gift from God, and the gift is differentially bestowed. Healing practitioners, that is, can be ranked according to how much "power" God has given them to cure. There

are three ranks of healers graded in this way, the lowest including those who learned their craft from others, whether one's grandmother, a talented neighbor, or a medical school—the M.D. or D.O., therefore, is classed along with the herb doctor and neighborhood healer. Above these are those individuals whom God thought fit to receive the gift of healing, during a religious experience later in life; evangelist Oral Roberts is a well-known example of this kind of healer. The individual with the greatest ability, however, is the person born with the gift of healing, which is evidence of special divine approbation literally from birth.[13]

The power of the spiritually gifted healer to offer divine deliverance is contrasted with the doctor's limited ability to heal serious diseases such as cancer:

See, now, if you have cancer, the doctors can't cure cancer! But if they go prayin' for you, and you have lots of faith, the Lord will cure that cancer! The Lord heals a whole lot of people of things the doctors done give up! While the doctor may give you up, the Lord can come in and deliver you! Put you on your feet! Then whenever the doctor come back and examine you for that particular thing and he don't see it, why, he'll say, "Well, I know it was there, but I don't know what became of you now!" They'll be amazed theirself; they want to know what happened![14]

Snow also documents the skepticism of many of the poor toward medicine and physicians by way of a succinct exclamation by an eighty-two-year-old woman who credited her long life and good health to the fact that she had always relied on her own herbal remedies: "My system ain't never been poisoned up by no medical doctor."[15]

This brief survey of Africans' and African Americans' beliefs and practices manifesting profound trust in the healing power of God illumines our understanding of the black postal workers' decision to reject medical treatment and "trust God." However, the testimony of mistrust in medicine, where staying away from doctors and medicine is viewed as the key to longevity and good health, further explains the attitudes and behavior of the black postal workers, especially when considered in light of the history of racist medical experimentation involving African Americans.

Black "Guinea Pigs" and the Problem of Race in American Medicine

When the black postal workers referred to themselves as "guinea pigs" in the course of deciding whether or not to accept medications and treatment in the wake of their exposure to anthrax, the term conjures two historical examples of blacks being used as "guinea pigs" in medical experimentation without regard for their increased risks of suffering or death. First is the gynecological experimentation of J. Marion Sims in the nineteenth century, and the second is the more widely known and well-documented Tuskegee Syphilis Study involving syphilitic black males in the twentieth century.

The cruel experimentation of Dr. J. Marion Sims using slave women is documented in the two-volume series *An American Health Dilemma: A Medical History of African Americans and the Problem of Race.* This ground-breaking study of the medical history of African Americans is written by two physicians, W. Michael Byrd and Linda A. Clayton. They analyze the hostility and contempt with which the medical profession has approached the health and healing of African Americans. Their careful documentation of the horrifying legacy of unethical experimentation on black human subjects in the nineteenth century is exemplified by Sims, known as the "father" of gynecology and vaginal surgery, who developed his techniques by operating on slave women, one of whom he purchased for the express purpose of performing experimental gynecological surgery on her: "He performed repeated major surgical procedures . . . exposing their genitals to the public, without anesthesia—believing Blacks did not have morals or perceive pain as Whites did. Moreover, to manipulate their postoperative healing process he addicted them to opiates (equivalent to morphine or heroin) to modulate their bowel and bladder function. Medical exploitation of the Black slaves was accepted without comment."[16] Sims admitted to operating on one slave woman at least thirty times.

Byrd and Clayton reveal the ironic conclusion drawn by American medical scientists studying the effects of emancipation on black health, that "freedom had caused the physical, moral, and mental degeneration of African Americans."[17] The prediction of black extinction by the year 2000 was developed on the authority of health-based statistical sources (including the eighth U.S. Census) and used to convince "most insurance companies by 1900 that Blacks were uninsurable."[18] Their summary of the phenomena manifesting the racist assumptions and practices of nineteenth-century medical science reads as a sweeping indictment of the American health care delivery system as measured by its treatment of blacks:

> the medical and scientific assumption of Black racial inferiority and "difference" from the rest of the human family; the assumption of poor and deteriorating Black health status and outcome as normal and inevitable; the belief that Black racial extinction, largely due to health causes, would occur in the twentieth century; the victim-blaming belief that the Black health crisis was the African American's fault; and the belief that a combination of health and social causes working against Blacks would ultimately solve the race problem in America by making the race extinct.[19]

As earlier chapters in this book have discussed, the more recent example familiar to many African Americans is the Tuskegee Syphilis Study, known also as the Tuskegee Experiment. Emilie Townes has included a chapter on this experiment in her 1998 book, *Breaking the Fine Rain of Death*. She explains that the Tuskegee Syphilis Study was conducted by the U.S. Public Health Service over a forty-year period, from 1932 to 1972. Four hundred black men in rural Macon County, Alabama, were diagnosed with syphilis and studied without being treated for the disease: "The [Public Health Service] did not tell these men that they had syphilis, and the service did not treat them so that researchers could discover the "natural history" of the disease. The end-point of the study was death, at which time the researchers autopsied the men to see what havoc the disease had wrought on their internal organs. Medical personnel never warned the men that they could pass the disease on to their sex partners or to their unborn children."[20]

The legacy of this experiment for African Americans is a profound and extensive sense of distrust of public health authorities, warranted by statements such as the following made by Dr. John Heller, director of Venereal Diseases at the Public Health Service from 1943 to 1948, in an interview conducted four years after the conclusion of the experiment, that "the men's status did not warrant ethical debate. They were subjects, not patients; clinical material, not sick people."[21] The federal government acknowledged the wrongs done and paid a $10 million settlement to the victims and their heirs in 1974. In 1997 President Bill Clinton issued a formal apology to the survivors of the study and their families and to the surviving family members of those men who had died.[22] The president announced the award of a $200,000 grant to Tuskegee University to initiate the National Center for Bioethics in Research and Health Care, and more than $20 million in grants and pledges were made to the university to help establish and operate the center.

Conclusion

The Brentwood postal facility was reopened on December 22, 2003, and re-named the Curseen-Morris Mail Processing and Distribution Center in memory of the two postal workers who died. It took twenty-two months and $130 million to complete the chlorine dioxide fumigation process and to replace contaminated office equipment, machinery, plumbing, and other fix-tures. However, the discussion and debate concerning the allegations of un-equal treatment and the use of postal workers as guinea pigs have by no means come to an end. On September 9, 2004, the United States Govern-ment Accountability Office (GAO) released a report of their review of the government's response to the anthrax contamination at five postal process-ing and distribution centers, including the Brentwood facility where the fatalities occurred. This report responds to a request from congressional leaders representing the affected districts: Senator Joseph I. Lieberman of Connecticut, Congressman Christopher H. Smith of New Jersey, and Eleanor Holmes Norton, delegate to Congress representing the District of Columbia. Four specific questions were investigated in the GAO report, each of which bears upon the problem of unequal treatment: (1) the factors considered in deciding whether to close the five facilities and the actions taken to protect postal employees; (2) the information communicated to affected postal em-ployees about the health risks posed by, and the extent of, contamination in the five facilities; (3) how lessons learned from the response to the contami-nation could be used in future situations; and (4) what, if any, medical ser-vices and reassignment benefits were provided to employees at the five fa-cilities and how these benefits compared across these facilities as well with those provided to employees at facilities closed for other emergencies be-tween January 1, 1998, and December 31, 2002.[23]

The GAO report analyzes the steps taken by the Postal Service and the CDC and attempts to explain how these actions contributed to the percep-tion of unequal treatment:

Public health agencies underestimated the health risks to postal em-ployees, in part, because they did not know that anthrax spores could leak from taped, unopened letters in sufficient quantities to cause a fatal form of anthrax. The Postal Service kept the three other facilities covered by GAO's review open because public health officials had advised the agency that employees at those centers were at minimal risk. CDC and the Postal Service have said they would have made different decisions if they had earlier understood the health risks to postal employees. The Postal Service communicated information to affected postal employees about the health risks posed by, and the extent of, anthrax contamination at the five facilities in GAO's review, but problems with accuracy, clarity, and timeliness led employees to question the information they received.[24]

The report also thoroughly explains the circumstances surrounding the postal workers' perception of themselves being used as guinea pigs:

CDC had to administer the vaccine using extensive protocols that the Food and Drug Administration requires for an "investigational new drug." These protocols, which are standard for new drugs, required postal employees to complete more paperwork and undergo more monitoring than for approved drugs. According to some postal employees, the protocols made them feel like "guinea pigs." CDC officials acknowledged that CDC did not explain the vaccine program clearly and concluded, in hindsight, that communication problems probably contributed to the misperceptions of postal employees and others potentially exposed to the disease.[25]

The GAO concludes that the dangerously delayed response to the anthrax contamination of postal facilities is attributable to the fact that public health officials underestimated the health risks involved. The most important lesson learned is somewhat obvious, that "agencies need to choose a course of action that poses the least risk of harm when considering actions to protect people from uncertain and potentially life-threatening health risks."[26] The challenge remains to find ways to ensure that such protections are extended equally to all persons, even in the face of uncertainty and grave danger.

I have argued that the black postal workers who expressed trust in God rather than in medicine or the government in response to the anthrax assault spoke and acted in harmony with the folk religion and historical memory of a people whose health has been unjustly disregarded and even damaged by unethical experimentation. As more policies and strategies are set forth by our government to secure our nation from further attacks, it is my hope that lessons learned from the experience and perspectives of the black postal workers will enhance our own best efforts to protect the well-being of all our citizens under ongoing conditions of extreme uncertainty and danger.

Notes

1. Avram Goldstein, "Many Postal Workers Stop Taking Cipro," *Washington Post*, December 10, 2001, p. B02.
2. Steve Twomey, "Vaccine Offer Draws Few Postal Workers," *Washington Post*, December 28, 2001, p. A06.
3. *Doctors for Disaster Preparedness Newsletter* 19 (March 2002). Retrieved November 29, 2006, from www.oism/org/ddp/ddpnews/ddpmar02.htm
4. Gerhardus C. Oosthuizen, *The Healer-Prophet in Afro-Christian Churches* (Leiden: E. J. Brill, 1992), 41.
5. Albert J. Raboteau, "The Afro-American Tradition," in Ronald L. Numbers and Darrel W. Amundsen, eds., *Caring and Curing: Health and Medicine in the Western Religious Traditions* (Baltimore, MD: Johns Hopkins University Press, 1998), 544.
6. Sharla Fett, "It's a Spirit in Me: Spiritual Power and the Healing Work of African American Women in Slavery," in *A Mighty Baptism*, ed. Susan Juster and Lisa MacFarlane (Ithaca, NY: Cornell University Press, 1996), 204.
7. Beverly J. Robinson, "Africanisms and the Study of Folklore," in *Africanisms in American Culture*, ed. Joseph E. Holloway (Bloomington: Indiana University Press, 1990), 218.
8. Fett, "It's a Spirit in Me," 193–97.
9. Ibid., 208.
10. Raboteau, "The Afro-American Tradition," 555.
11. Ibid.
12. Grant Wacker, "The Pentecostal Tradition," in *Caring and Curing: Health and Medicine in the Western Religious Traditions*, ed. Ronald L. Numbers and Darrel W. Amundsen (Baltimore: Johns Hopkins University Press, 1998), 524.
13. Loudell F. Snow, "Folk Medical Beliefs and Their Implications for Care of Patients: A Review Based on Studies among Black Americans," *Annals of Internal Medicine* 81 (1974): 93.
14. Quoted in ibid, 94n: Arnelia L., Tucson, Arizona, age 64, born Texas, sixth-grade education. Excerpt from tape recording, January 1971.

15. Loudell F. Snow, "Traditional Health Beliefs and Practices among Lower Class Black Americans," *Western Journal of Medicine* 139 (December 1983): 821.

16. W. Michael Byrd and Linda A. Clayton, *An American Health Dilemma: A Medical History of African Americans and the Problem of Race, Beginnings to 1900* (New York: Routledge, 2000), 273–74.

17. Ibid., 410.

18. Ibid., 411.

19. Ibid., 412.

20. Emilie M. Townes, *Breaking the Fine Rain of Death: African American Health Issues and a Womanist Ethic of Care* (New York: Continuum, 1998), 88.

21. Stephen B. Thomas and Sandra Crouse Quinn, "The AIDS Epidemic and the African American Community: Toward an Ethical Framework for Service Delivery," in *It Just Ain't Fair: The Ethics of Health Care for African Americans*, ed. Annette Dula and Sara Goering (Westport, CT: Praeger, 1994), 83.

22. Townes, *Breaking the Fine Rain of Death*, 100.

23. GAO, "U.S. Postal Service: Better Guidance Is Needed to Ensure an Appropriate Response to Anthrax Contamination," GAO-04-239 (Washington, DC: U.S. Government Accountability Office, September 9, 2004), 2–3.

24. In ibid., "Highlights."

25. Ibid., 31–32.

26. In ibid., "Highlights."

CHAPTER 6

Personal Narrative and an African American Perspective on Medical Ethics

Ezra E. H. Griffith

B I O M E D I C A L ethics is a subject that is attracting much attention both from laypersons and from health care professionals. Indeed, I believe that developments in other peripherally related areas are catalyzing this renewed general interest in ethics. The Abu Ghraib prison debacle in Iraq certainly has contributed to focusing attention on the ethics of prosecuting war. But it is the possible direct or indirect involvement of physicians in the activity of torture that has furthered greater interest in the ethics of health care professionals.[1] Other revelations have now suggested that the medical records of detainees at Guantanamo Bay, Cuba, have been made available to interrogators and those torturing the detainees.[2] What medical professionals do, or don't do, is of current interest to us all. Everybody wants to know how the medical professional develops and articulates a moral foundation on which to base a way of leading his or her professional life.

Of course, this curiosity and interest are not new. They have just been, once again, reawakened by the discovery of the conditions at Abu Ghraib and Guantanamo Bay. And while some would have us believe that those conditions reflect an unusual and aberrant context, commentators such as Lifton remind us that any one of us, including physicians, can be caught in an "atrocity-producing situation."[3] By that, Lifton meant that it was possible for doctors to be socialized to atrocity by being exposed to a context that was structured psychologically and administratively to facilitate commission of atrocities. While Lifton was preoccupied in his earlier work with doctors of the Nazi regime, he certainly noted that American physicians, like anybody else, could be exposed to institutional pressures that might lead them to violate their consciences. This leads inexorably back to the question of how medical professionals construct the moral foundations of their professional lives. It is an intriguing question, and I shall dwell on it in this chapter, although with emphasis on how black physicians accomplish it. However, given my intellectual interest in narrative and memoir, I have decided to concentrate first on a longitudinal exposition about the constructing of the moral foundation undergirding my professional life. For my narrative to make sense, I note that I am a member of the nondominant black group in the United States, and my professional identity is that of a forensic psychiatrist.

I resort to telling a brief story about my life, not only because I am preparing a terrain of argument that will highlight a stark preference for narrative ethics but also because I do not think it easy to articulate my own African American perspective on biomedical ethics without outlining some personal experiences that have contributed to the shaping of my moral life. These experiences will be notably religious and cultural, which may immediately evoke sympathy from philosophers and scientists about the parochial nature of my background. Nevertheless, that is the way it is. I cannot invent another version of my longitudinal, psychosocial development. So, in sharpening my intent, I should say that I wish to focus on the pathways used by me, a black physician and forensic psychiatry specialist, to construct the moral foundation of my professional identity. I shall ultimately apply my argumentation to a current debate on the ethics of forensic psychiatry practice.

Background

Early one morning in the 1940s, my father sent the usual message to the midwife who had served our family before. I understand she arrived and performed her duties effectively. As a consequence, I first saw the light of day in a small chattel house located in the Caribbean island of Barbados. In those days, that lovely piece of territory was a British possession, one of those outlying countries that the British Colonial Office followed attentively.

I was raised amidst the multiple paradoxes that so traditionally characterized life in the British Empire. On the one hand, I received a solid education at the levels of primary and secondary school. I read widely and engaged in critical discourse with teachers and friends. Indeed, debate of all topics was a hallowed part of Barbadian culture. On the other hand, I came to understand that the British saw themselves in a different light from the way they viewed those they colonized. As a result, I internalized the metaphor of the club—in this case, the aquatic club and the yacht club. To their credit, the British did not put up signs saying that black Barbadians could not use the two clubs. As I have stated elsewhere,[4] the British did not engage in such gauche behavior. Nevertheless, the unwritten rule that I was to stay away was as clear to me as any regulation could be to people with common sense. So I went to neither club. In subsequent years, I began to appreciate more acutely this idea that black people were accorded privileges that were different from ones enjoyed by whites. And it would unleash in me a preoccupation with this distinction between dominant and nondominant groups.

The subtlety of the British is ineffaceable in my mind. I saw it at work even in the church context, and I marveled at their technique. For several years I sang in the choir of the local Anglican Cathedral; I was a part of the age-old British tradition of boy choristers. So I sang both at the Sunday morning matins service and at the seven o'clock evensong. I could never understand why the white Britishers had a preference for the morning service. Few were present at the evening service. This resulted in a peculiar separation of the black and white groups that helped me to formulate an understanding of difference in the British colonial context. It didn't take me long to note that few bank tellers were black or that the head of this organization and the leader of that association were white.

When, in 1956, my family moved to the United States, another phase of my sociopolitical education began. It was around this time that I first read Richard Wright's *Native Son*[5] and confronted such raw anger spilling from a writer's pen. This was years before the formulation of African American studies, and I had to take responsibility for my own intellectual development. I cannot even remember what led me to read about the Harlem Renaissance. But I know it was not in formal courses anywhere that I encountered the term. It would be just after my graduation from college in 1963 that I heard Malcolm X give a lecture in Boston, saw him field questions expertly, spouting back rhetoric that frightened both blacks and whites. In those days, many of the people I knew wanted to find some ground for accommodation, for compromise. Only a few people in my circle wanted a revolution, a Baldwinian fire, or a Rap Brownian burning. But most of my friends did want change. After all, it was time for things to improve everywhere for blacks.

Without extending the story anymore, I realized that many of my social and intellectual experiences sensitized me to the peculiar context of the Anglo-American world. I learned that there was a dominant white group and a nondominant black group, and the interactions between the two groups were complicated, often abrasive, and pervasively contentious. (This is not to suggest that there are not other nondominant groups, or that the only way to think about dominant and nondominant group interaction is on the basis of skin color. However, for purposes of simplicity, I will limit my attention here to the exchanges of whites and blacks.)

I turn now to the other important dimension of my early social experiences both in Barbados and in the United States. These experiences took place in the church. I use the term *church* in a broad Protestant sense and without reference either to the Catholic religion or to Jewish dogma. I attended many different churches, as a result more of geographic convenience than any intended philosophical distinctiveness. But over time, I progressively came to see the church as a means of thinking about social justice, of reflecting on the plight of the poor, and as a mechanism for facilitating the interaction of dominant and nondominant groups based on fairness and equity.

At this juncture, I am not insisting that any black individual growing up in the Anglo-American world would have or should have reached the same conclusions that I reached. We are all more sophisticated now than a decade ago, and we know that members of nondominant groups are capable of formulating different approaches to their problems and to the articulating of solutions. But I decided that in the Anglo-American context, most of my acts are viewed as the movements of a black man and weighed on scales ultimately controlled by nonblacks. It saddens me, too, that simply because of my membership in a nondominant, nonwhite group, I spend considerable energy preoccupied with the task of living my life as a black individual. I reflect incessantly on the interaction of blacks and whites. Why? Simply because skin color matters in this country, and racism, its derivative, is a pollutant that taints black-white interactions. Furthermore, black responses to the white dominant group are so complicated that the problem of responding strategically to whites is, in my view, a lifelong task within Levinson's scheme.[6] When Levinson articulated his theory of life cycle stages, he assigned major tasks to each phase of life. For example, we understand now how a recent college graduate of about twenty-one years old looks to the work of defining an early direction for his or her career and simultaneously struggles to establish a life that is set off from that of the parents. But Levinson never explicitly enunciated this task that I think is so important for blacks in this particular cultural setting of the United States. In all fairness, he understood it—something that was clear in the many discussions that I had with him before his death. In addition, he was quite sensitive to the tasks of women, and he understood that the symbol of nondominant/dominant group interactions had wider applicability than only to the dichotomous pair of black/white.

I wish to assert, and to do so more strenuously and energetically than Levinson, that black individuals do well to face the objective of measuring and even trying to control their interactions with whites. I make no bones about my special interest in how black professionals—in this case, psychiatrists—prosecute the task. I intend to offer the outline of an approach to contending with this objective, which in my mind is almost synonymous with what I consider to be a duty of professionals from nondominant groups. The approach requires that black professionals, for example, reflect earnestly on how they authentically represent their nondominant group. They must also consider the phenomena of "belonging" and of "nigrescence building." These three elements are powerful forces that impinge on the way black psychiatrists do their work and think about their lives. These forces also lead to a unique forging of an ethics-based platform on which to carry out one's professional activity. I would like to render this process clearer and more palpable, thereby making it more readily understandable.

However, before moving on, I underline a point I made earlier. It is often expected that all those assigned to a particular nondominant group have a common way of viewing the world and that they accommodate to a clearly defined way of dealing with dominant group members. In a broad sense, that is why so many of us find it hard to understand that the black individual who defines himself as a conservative Republican is even conceptually possible as a definitional entity. But we certainly know now that black conservative Republicans exist. They are alive and functioning well and intent on growing in number. This means that the task of adapting to the dominant white group is open to interpretational adjustment, regardless of what our own personal preferences may be. This is why I prefer to emphasize comprehension of the problem and leave the question of stylized choice to each individual. This does not mean I have no preference. I just recognize that others may not like my preference. My point is, therefore, that I want us to agree with Gates's idea that the notion of a unitary black man is but an imaginary concept.[7] Hence the interest in my own narrative as a point of departure. There is some recognition then of the reality that every black man has his own gauntlet to run.

Authentic Representation

I turn now to the problem of authentic representation, which I point out is a special burden for black psychiatrists, although I have already conceded that, generally speaking, members of nondominant groups must come to terms with the task of authentically representing their group. But clear understanding of the task requires its own deconstruction. So I shall deal first with representation.

The burden of representing one's nondominant black group has, for a long time, been a prominent theme in the cultural context of the United States. Race men such as W. E. B. Du Bois and Booker T. Washington understood it well. In Sister Souljah's autobiography titled *No Disrespect*, she noted that Harriet Tubman "could have just chilled in the North, built a white house with a white picket fence, got a light-skinned husband and died with her fingertips in a jar of skin-lightening cream. But she didn't. She marched her big black ass through the woods . . . and went back and got her African brothers and sisters."[8]

Now this quotation is somewhat provocative, as Sister Souljah is wont to be. So for a bit, I suggest we look past the provocation of the comfortable white house, the light-skinned husband, and the skin-lightening cream. And no matter! We are still left with Sister Souljah's insistence that we make a commitment to help save our brothers and sisters from the injustices and indignities meted out by members of the dominant white group. We must, therefore, represent them and not sit comfortably ensconced in whatever luxury our economic achievement will purchase for us. Others such as Chester Pierce[9] have raised the question in a more subdued but still penetrating tone: How will you serve the group, the nondominant group that so lucidly contributes at least partly to the establishment of your identity in this country?

Now when we return to the rest of Sister Souljah's passage, we see that she articulates a polarized view of representation. After all, Harriet Tubman could have built herself a white house, found a light-skinned husband, dug deeply into the skin-lightening cream, and still marched back through the woods for her brothers and sisters. For the sake of argument, one could serve the group and still adhere to personalized concepts that may even seem to be at odds with one's service to the group. So I place Sister Souljah, partly for pragmatic didactic purposes, at one polar end of a spectrum of possibilities.

At the other end comes what Henry Louis Gates calls soulless, colorless opportunism.[10] That depiction speaks by and for itself. That end of the spectrum makes no pretenses about representing anybody. That is the plea for being just a human being and leaving the burden of representing to others. At this end of the spectrum, the salience of race or ethnicity is minimal, if not nonexistent.

Between those two poles on the spectrum reside a host of stylized roads to representing the black nondominant group. If I understand what Cross has to say about the complexity of developing both personal and group black identity, I expect that there is often ambivalence in us blacks about representing our constituency.[11] So that while we are representing, we may also be rebelling against the very task. This explains Gates's joke about blacks' being embarrassed by another black who is too dark, too loud, and too wrong. "Nigger is loud and wrong," Gates would say.[12] And the unstated question is who wants to represent someone like that.

Now Gates put his finger quite naturally on another special problem that educated, nondominant group members like us must have. Our education, experience, and socialization as physicians and psychiatrists make it easy for us to engage in what Gates calls the constructing of "identities through elective affinity."[13] So, for example, we play golf and hang around with golfers. As we participate in this endeavor, skin color is not an important characteristic. It allows us, in Gates's terms, to "experience a humanity that is neither colorless nor reducible to color."[14] Now what I intended to show here is the marvelous array of options presented to the black psychiatrist who contemplates the task of representing his nondominant group.

Obviously, the pervasive and extensive establishment of elective affinities can lead to one's adopting the stance of colorless opportunism. I need not criticize that preference, to which some black professionals naturally gravitate. Suffice it to say that some blacks contemplate the burden of representation, define it as too heavy and costly a burden, and then move to activities where the salience of race matters is minimal. In my own case, I have adopted a clearly personal form of representation in my private and professional life. This I have done as a function of my background and narrative experience. But, in addition, the salience of skin color is unambiguous in the areas of my professional interests: medicine and the law.[15]

I do wish to make explicit an idea that I assume others may have. I never intended to suggest that members of the dominant white group do not engage in the process of representation. Such a thought is to my mind preposterous. However, little effort is needed to point out that representing the dominant group must be a qualitatively different matter from representing a nondominant group. That, after all, is at the heart of understanding what difference and hierarchical difference are all about when we talk of dominant and nondominant groups.

First of all, except in the rare situation where dominant group membership is significantly smaller than nondominant group membership or in the unusual context where nondominant group members have become overtly rebellious and violent, dominant group members enjoy the luxury of avoiding reflection on the task of representing. Of course, they may enjoy engaging in representation of the values they hold dear. Some years ago, when the Black Panthers attacked dominant group values with a certain vehemence and then went on to threaten violence, dominant group members became palpably terrified and even moved to the task of representing the dominant group with unaccustomed vigor.

However, for the most part, the members of dominant groups do not have to gear their style of representing to anticipated responses from the nondominant group. The dominant group is taken with superiority and the image of spreading their ideas to others. In a few words, I dare say that the burden of representing a dominant group and doing it from what I shall call a "one-up position" must be qualitatively different from the task of representing a nondominant group from a "one-down position." This distinction is perhaps most movingly articulated in Linda Brent's slave narrative *Incidents in the Life of a Slave Girl*.[16] There, Dr. Flint, the slave master, certainly rises to the task of effectively representing the group of autocratic slave owners. And he demonstrated that the dominant group can also take on the burden of representation. Consequently, he takes a certain vindictive pleasure in asserting his role as slave master and seeking to bend Linda Brent's will to his as he tries, and I say it in modern-day parlance, to get into her pants. It was the good doctor's view that both Linda and her pants belonged to him. With all of that said, I concede that dominant group representation may well be a function of how vigorously the opposing nondominant group represents itself. So the luxury of dominant group representation may not always be as pronounced as nondominant group members imagine.

Authenticity

I come now to the dimension of authenticity, which I argue adds more weight to the burden of representation. This notion of authenticity exerts a distinct pressure on the act of representing. It pulls the nondominant group individual in a particular direction and adds a special patina to the process of representation. If we return quickly to Sister Souljah's characterization of Harriet Tubman, we must understand why Sister Souljah insisted that Harriet Tubman did not build a white house with a picket fence and that Ms. Tubman also gave up the light-skinned husband and the jar of skin-lightening cream. In other words, Ms. Tubman not only bore the burden of representing her nondominant group brethren, she did so authentically. Sister Souljah has no hesitation in adding to the burden.

The insistence on the authentic prosecution of representation comes most forcefully at times from other members of our nondominant group. That is why nondominant group members enjoy the juxtaposing of our heroes: Jesse Jackson and Colin Powell, Martin Luther King and Malcolm X, James Baldwin and Eldridge Cleaver, Clarence Thomas and Leon Higginbotham. The juxtapositioning makes us confront our own fears. In each pair, we see stylized representing. Both individuals can be easily linked to the work of representing the nondominant black group. But one of them is doing so more authentically than the other, although we may all differ on who is the authentic one. There is no empirical basis on which to make my claim, but my repeated conversations with psychiatrist colleagues and other black professionals have persuaded me that they are unduly preoccupied with carrying the burden of representation. They also dread the potential accusation that they are pursuing their representation inauthentically, which I see as proximate to a charge of treason, of betrayal. That is why I think it's so important for minority professionals to settle in their minds what they conclusively feel is authentic representation.

Not surprisingly, of course, the situation is often rendered more complicated when members of the dominant group enter the fray and try to add their two bits to a discussion that nondominant group members often see as no business at all of the dominant group. I have tried on numerous occasions to explain this to white colleagues, and they have always appeared nonplussed and confused at my explanation. I point out to them that in the trial of *United States v. Marion Barry*, many African Americans were offended by the uniquely vicious way in which the authorities hounded Mayor Barry. African Americans were offended too by the suggestion, which was implicit in the government's charges, that the mayor had represented his constituents inauthentically. In other words, the mayor had not served his black brothers and sisters well. But many blacks thought that whites were intent on imposing their views on Barry's black constituents.

This subject of authentic representation remains a topic of cardinal significance at least because it invokes the use of so much energy in its contemplation. But it is important also because it influences the way in which black professionals decide to live out their lives and to construct the moral base on which the professional orientation is founded. Lithwick's critique of the recent biography of Clarence Thomas raises the fundamental question of how could a black man "who filters each and every public sling and arrow he's suffered through the prism of his own victimization construct for himself a jurisprudence of disdain for victims?"[17] It's another way of asking how to move from Thomas's personal narrative to his professional credo. What is clearly missing in Thomas's story is the element articulated by Lawrence-Lightfoot in her portraiture of black men and women—that they are "courageous in pursuing their dreams and in reconciling with their roots."[18] It is this reconciliation with Thomas's roots that was of interest to Higginbotham, who rephrased the question another way. Higginbotham wanted to know how, given Justice Thomas's background, Thomas could formulate the moral basis to become hostile to affirmative action opportunities.[19] Higginbotham therefore made the connection between personal narrative and the moral construction of one's professional life, to which I shall subsequently return.

Belonging and Nigrescence Building

The metaphor of belonging refers to a developmental process that I shall describe shortly. Much like the burden of representation, working out the difficulties presented by the belonging process may take many years, and it extends across the life span. The process of belonging may be understood as a correlative activity to the constructing of one's racial identity attitudes, what Thomas Parham[20] and William Cross[21] have labeled a process of psychological nigrescence.

What is meant by the phenomenon of belonging? Belonging has been described as a total and confident sense of being a member of an organization.[22] It is markedly different from the feeling of being tolerated or, worse, the feeling that you are an uninvited guest, a party crasher, so to speak. It is even different from the feeling that you have worked hard to get there and deserve the opportunity to be there. This sense of belonging is also more than mere confidence. When you really have the feeling of belonging, you don't waste time wondering what some white individual meant, who only apparently slighted you; you don't constantly look around trying to gauge your effect on the white people around you. You pursue your activities with efficient single-mindedness, mindful of the need to be gracious and respectful of others. When you belong, you move with grace and aplomb. You contribute to setting the tone of the interaction when dealing with your white peers, and you know the limits of what you will accept from your white superiors. To those less fortunate than you, you are always patient and helpful. This sense of belonging is definitely more than just confidence.

It is perhaps better explicated through the description of how a black belongs to a black institution. The black who "belongs" to his church is totally at ease with all the rituals. His knowledge of the rules constrains him only a little. And while parameters are set that influence thinking and behavior, his creativity is often enhanced. The black who "belongs" to his church will testify, pray out loud, fall in the Spirit. He has no hesitation in saying "Amen" out loud or in clapping and laughing when he wishes. He feels in control of his space and time and knows with absolute certainty that it is his church. In fact, he alters his behavior when he visits another church, even if he has good friends there, because that is not his home church. His belonging isn't just psychological or social. It has physical and behavioral correlates that are reflected in his total deportment.

It should be emphasized that when an individual does not belong somewhere, he spends an inordinate amount of energy thinking about what the dominant group intends doing to him or about what the dominant group thinks of him. This is what Chester Pierce called "defensive, apologetic, and deferential" thinking,[23] which leads to relative paralysis of his action and planning. In turn, this impacts on his self-esteem and effectiveness. Running away from the contentiousness of the dominant/nondominant interaction is not expected to be helpful in the long run. The important task is for members of the nondominant group to learn how to negotiate the interactions with the dominant group and emerge with their self-esteem intact and elevated.

I come full circle now to Sara Lawrence-Lightfoot's *I've Known Rivers*.[24] In her analysis of six black lives, she drew attention to Harvard's Professor Ogletree and his continuing question about whether he should be exercising his functions at a place like Harvard. Even those who apparently made it in the white-dominated marketplace seem unable to resolve effectively the complex struggle of being at peace with their membership in white-dominated organizations. Professor Ogletree, at least in the skilled portraiture hands of Lawrence-Lightfoot, comes across as a wonderful example of the problematic intermingling of the belonging process and the burden of representation. The professor is taken with the idea that his feeling comfortable and ultimately belonging at Harvard may dilute his capacity to represent his black brothers and sisters effectively.

Cross,[25] in his early theorizing, suggested several phases of identity development, which Parham[26] illustrated later with attention to the narratives of Malcolm X and W. E. B. Du Bois. With reference to Malcolm X, for example, Parham explained how in the "Pre-encounter stage," Malcolm was a high school adolescent who had little feeling about the business of being a black man. Then in the "Encounter" stage, Malcolm has his famous experience with the English teacher who tells Malcolm that being a lawyer is no realistic goal for a nigger. At that point, Malcolm begins to be more contemplative whenever he hears the word *nigger*. In his "Immersion-Emersion" stage, Malcolm begins to read voraciously whatever he can find in the prison library about black history. It is then that he is converted to the Muslim lifestyle. In his "Internalization" phase, Malcolm is on the pilgrimage to Mecca and encounters Muslims of different races. He begins then to reevaluate his perceptions about white men, and by extension, rethinks his views of the interactions between members of the nondominant black group and members of the dominant white group in the United States.

Parham also made the point that a black individual's movement from one state to the next, and often back again, is influenced by experiences with both whites and blacks. In addition, movement through the nigrescence process is a function too of the Levinsonian state at which nigrescence experiences occur. Parham further emphasized that any black individual may proceed through Cross's nigrescence process in a stagewise linear fashion; one may also stagnate or recycle through the process. What is most crucial to understand, however, is that one's style of adapting to the nigrescence or belonging process ultimately may shape one's professional work.

Constructing a Moral Foundation

Up to now I have tried to expose the powerful forces that impinge repeatedly on black medical professionals in the course of their work. But I do not wish to be seen as encouraging disordered thinking and behavior among physicians who belong to the nondominant groups of this country. In other words, I am not promoting chaos. However, I knew no other way to focus on the mission of creating an exposition of how I am struggling to do my professional work, without articulating a narrative of my experiences. Furthermore, it is my view that my personal story is starkly defined by my identity as a black professional. Gates has asserted that nobody happens to be black,[27] and it is a definitional truth that flies in the face of the comforting old lie that I could be a professional who happens to be black. However, I reject the comfort and the untruth because they serve no purpose in my argumentation. I turn now to my reality, which is founded on the precept that in constructing a moral foundation for my work, I have had to take stock of the burden of authentic representation and of the phenomena of belonging and nigrescence.

I am aware, after having carefully reviewed recent work about African American perspectives on biomedical ethics,[28] that there is a difference of opinion as to whether one can claim a unique black approach to the constructing of a moral platform on which to found one's medical work. Obviously, each professional must reach his own opinion. However, I am concerned that black professionals may indeed find it easier to voice opinions about the moral context of their work by expressing themselves in a way that may still strategically serve the interests of the dominant group, what Sampson calls an accommodative voice.[29] It is a way of thinking about morality and ethics, but within the parameters of dominant-group discourse. In resorting to personal narrative, I seek to broker a position that I hope is transformative: I have tried to articulate my own constitutive reality, keeping it real as I feel it to be, and then making it clear that the development and orientation of my own identity have influenced my effort to formulate self-determining self-representation. Consequently, my morality is harnessed to my narrative background.

Let us now examine a specific ethics dilemma I have encountered in my practice of forensic psychiatry, which is a unique specialty branch of

117

clinical medicine. Because forensic psychiatric work takes place at the nexus of psychiatry and the law, the activities are often broader than those of traditional clinical psychiatry and therefore may create problematic situations that are somewhat unusual in clinical medicine.

Professor Alan Stone framed this particular dilemma some years ago, and he started by recounting an aged story, one that rightly deserves to be called a parable, because once he has related the story, Stone went on to deduce from it a range of powerful arguments. Stone gave the account of a Jewish physician who went to a British court in 1801 to help with the defense of another Jew who had stolen some spoons. At cross-examination, the prosecutor asked Dr. Leo: "Have you not been here before as a witness and a Jew physician, to give an account of a prisoner as a madman, to get him off upon the ground of insanity?"[30]

Given the relatively primitive knowledge of psychiatry at the time of Dr. Leo's testimony, Stone felt justified in asking whether Dr. Leo could have been in court to do anything else other than to help a fellow Jew escape just punishment. In other words, Dr. Leo was merely twisting justice and fairness to help his patient, the result of which was a desecration of his profession. Stone used the tale to examine the reference points or the ethics framework available to good Dr. Leo. Stone pointed out that, given the knowledge base of psychiatry at the time, neither a good clinical practice standard nor a scientific standard would have been of much use to Dr. Leo, who obviously knew little about his patient's "mania" for stealing spoons. Stone implicitly suggested, therefore, that Dr. Leo was lured into the courtroom by his wish to save his patient, to help his patient, which is in the tradition of clinicians. However, it is this desire to help, the "ethical thesis of the practitioner"[31] that became for Stone a fundamental problem in the legal context. Wishing to help leads the forensic psychiatrist into the temptation of going too far in his court testimony, of twisting things to help his patient. The result is ambiguity in the ethics boundaries of forensic psychiatry. The conclusion that flows from Stone's argumentation is that psychiatrists should stay out of the courtroom.

Appelbaum took Stone's criticism to heart and responded by delineating a theory of ethics for forensic psychiatry. Appelbaum was careful to define forensic psychiatry as the evaluation of subjects for the purpose of generating a report or testimony for an administrative or legal process.[32] In so doing, he sought to differentiate ethics principles as a function of the activities carried out by physicians. For Appelbaum, while beneficence toward his patient is a cardinal duty of a clinical doctor, a research physician may have an important commitment to the "production of valid, generalizable data."[33] Similarly, he saw forensic psychiatrists as having a commitment to the value of advancing justice, not to promoting the health of a patient. In advancing justice, Appelbaum argued that the forensic psychiatrist should focus squarely on truth telling and on maintaining respect for persons. Telling the truth requires saying what one believes to be true (a kind of honesty), as well as articulating the limitations on one's testimony (such as acknowledging clearly what records one has not seen). Respect for persons involves making clear to evaluation subjects the role being played by the physician, obtaining informed consent, and respecting confidentiality. Appelbaum did not dispense with a physician's duty to respect the traditional values of beneficence and nonmaleficence. However, he emphasized that those traditional values were not primarily relevant to carrying out the functions of a forensic psychiatrist.

So far, I have tried to explicate a major debate that has erupted in forensic psychiatry ethics, fueled especially by the arguments presented by Stone and the counterarguments formulated by Appelbaum. Elsewhere I responded to both colleagues and tried to establish what I found so unsatisfying about their positions.[34] First, I think it helpful and instructive to return briefly to Dr. Leo's story, as I have concluded that this Jewish physician is an important symbol of the nondominant group forensic psychiatrist. Dr. Leo had to confront his burden of representation. And given the anti-Semitic context at that time, he had to contemplate what commitment to his nondominant group could mean, what would be his behavior as he sought to represent his group authentically. I also cannot say where he was in Cross's framework of adult development and how his Jewish identity building was linked to his decision.

Nevertheless, what has made me increasingly troubled with the considerations evinced by both Stone and Appelbaum is how unconcerned they seemed with the profound dilemma faced by Dr. Leo. Stone seemed almost joyful at the idea that modern-day psychiatrists should stay out of the courtroom, given the ethics confusion pervading the work of forensic specialists. Furthermore, Appelbaum seemed to decide that truth telling and respect for persons would effectively serve all future Dr. Leos.

I can readily see that many colleagues will take up this last point and brandish it with fervor. In other words, Dr. Leo should forget his Jewishness and his struggles with dominant-group politics and simply tell the truth in the courtroom. This would solve a number of problems and should lead at least to striving for objectivity in his testimony. While I will ultimately dismiss this argument, I will not do so prematurely. Indeed, I pause here to amplify the point. In preparing this chapter, I took the time to review it with several colleagues. One of them, a black pastor, suggested that Dr. Leo was wrong in approaching the dilemma the way he did. The pastor suggested that Dr. Leo should not have been swayed by ethnicity or socioeconomic status, and Dr. Leo should have been committed to the universal principles of justice and truth telling. As a result, my pastor-colleague did not believe in leniency for minority groups and felt it unnecessary for them to be afforded a crutch or special helping hand. In his own language, he noted that he would recommend no breaching of the rules.

It surprised me how willing my colleague was to concede that blacks had had a terrible history in the Anglo-American context. Furthermore, he agreed that the current socioeconomic system was not fair to blacks. Neither were the legal and educational systems. He thought that Dr. Leo should have been constrained to tell the truth in court, while advocating outside the courtroom for equity and fairness for his nondominant group peers. My colleague then resorted to his religion-based terrain. He recommended a stance of "patient enduring," of "perseverance and hard work" for blacks throughout the Diaspora, and he described his hopeful belief that eventually blacks will be victorious in seeking equality and justice.

I have just pointed out how one religious colleague prized the value of truth telling and similar professional values. Even within a religious framework, this profound respect of such universal principles was desirable and important to maintain. Alternatively, another colleague (also a member of the cloth) pointed out that Dr. Leo deserved to be commended for the interest in his fellow man. Dr. Leo had an interest in the situation of his friends and neighbors, a sort of prophetic attachment to the orphan and the widow. Dr. Leo was responding to the injunction that we be concerned about feeding the hungry, clothing the naked, giving drink to the thirsty, and visiting those who are sick and in prison. My colleague saw Dr. Leo's behavior as, in a sense, imitative of Christ, calling to mind Christ's notion (found in St. Matthew's Gospel at 25:40) that "in as much as ye have done it unto one of the least of these my brethren, ye have done it unto me." (While I have formulated this idea in Christian terms, I recognize that other religions also preach compassion for one's neighbors.)

The juxtaposing of these religion-based views serves an important purpose. It highlights the crucial situational dilemma in which Dr. Leo found himself. And I am insisting that we must do right by Dr. Leo before blithely entertaining a solution. We must do better at understanding who Dr. Leo is. Dismissing the seriousness of his struggle is to undermine the personal narrative of nondominant group professionals. By dint of my own story and experience, I am forced to keep an eye on the interests of my nondominant group, even as I contemplate the values exhorted and underlined by my profession. Christ's injunction in the Gospel makes Dr. Leo a more sympathetic figure to my Christian mind and amplifies Dr. Leo's concern for his fellow Jew.

It worries me that one could observe Appelbaum's rules of truth telling and respect for persons without having any concern for the person who stole the spoons. At the same time, Dr. Leo could be concerned about his fellow Jew and go on to tell untruths and make false claims in court. The real task is to observe Appelbaum's principles while appreciating Christ's reminder about our interconnectedness. I am simply not satisfied by observing Appelbaum's rules in court, while the judicial system continues to be viewed by many as an institution pervasively plagued by racism.[35] Candilis and colleagues have also recognized that a tenacious respect for these ethics principles, with emphasis on objectivity, may lead to a less than humane consideration of our societal and professional obligations.[36]

As a black forensic psychiatrist, I am concerned about the commitment to professional values as well as about my self-defined loyalty to my reference group and my responsibility to others in my community. As a result, I take a transformative stance, wishing to advocate for adherence to professional values in addition to arguing forcefully for considering why Leo's group feels so disadvantaged and lacking empowerment. This approach also broadens and strengthens the business of respecting persons.

There are practical implications to this move. Ignoring my personal narrative diminishes me in my own eyes. But it also leads to minimizing of my group's status in the context of professional association politics. The result, as Cross understood so well,[37] often leads to an obligatory refurbishing of the process of nigrescence building. Rendering invisible a personal narrative can be perceived as, in Cross's terms, an unpleasant encounter experience, which in turn catalyzes a recycling through the nigrescence process. In other words, nonattention to Dr. Leo's dilemma can dilute the confidence that links him to his reference group, while making fragile his personal identity. I am also concerned that dominant group psychiatrists, some of whom spend little time reflecting on the situation of their nondominant group colleagues, often pursue with enthusiastic single-mindedness the political interests of the dominant group in the context of our professional organizations.

Now, I am not advocating commission of a wrong to correct an antecedent wrong. But I think it important and useful to advocate our participating differently in the work we do. First, we should approach the work while sensitively recognizing the pain and suffering of the defendants and others we are called to evaluate—owning them as one of us. In recognizing their status, we should work hard to make sure we do not exacerbate their suffering, although in some cases it may be unavoidable.

As we recognize the position of the disadvantaged in our midst and connect to them empathically, we must take on the responsibility to carry out our work as thoroughly as possible. It is in thinking more carefully about our evaluations—employing data from multiple sources when possible, emphasizing the need for completing the cultural formulation, checking and rechecking information—that we will do justice to the tasks we are hired to carry out. In other words, connecting to our subjects as human beings drives us to do our work professionally and humanely.

From time to time, those who represent the legal system will do their best to involve us in biased evaluations that harm or benefit the evaluee. It should be easy to resist the entreaties of those intent on harming. It will be harder to reject the invitation to twist what we have to say so as to benefit our subjects. Resisting this latter temptation is feasible if the expert is able to say that he or she is really committed to participating in a judicial process that is founded on fairness and an effort to provide justice to those caught up in it. However, the emphasis here is not on a platitudinous commitment to theoretical principles of truth telling and respect for persons. The emphasis is on a commitment to serving our neighbors fairly and respectfully—seeing them as members of our community and serving them as brothers and sisters.

Reflecting on the humanity in Dr. Leo's deportment has persuaded me that it is important to ask about the intent of those who wish to hire us. For example, some years ago a prosecutor hired me in the case of an individual who had refused to pay income taxes owed the government. I found out by accident that the prosecutor intended to pursue the case regardless of what I found on examining the subject. In other words, the prosecutor was not seeking justice. He simply intended to prosecute anyone who refused to pay taxes, and he confirmed that his was a political agenda. Many years later, I regret having taken the case. I did strive for objectivity in the case and pursued truth telling. I concluded that the subject suffered from a mental illness and that his thinking was delusional. But I did not think enough about the subject's humanity.

One final point: I am persuaded that our work takes on a different tone when truth telling, respect for persons, and objectivity are leavened with humanity and generosity. After concluding, for example, that a criminal defendant's state of mind has not reached the level of legal insanity, it helps to ask whether the defendant suffered from extreme emotional disturbance at the time of the crime or was able to form the requisite intent necessary for prosecution of the crime.

This is not twisting facts to help the defendant. It is acknowledging that the defendant is a person like me, a recognition that induces me into redoubling efforts to make sure I have done my work thoroughly. Understanding that the defendant is among "the least of these my brethren" argues for greater sustained consideration of how I am going about my work.

Notes

I thank Michael Norko, M.D., John Young, M.D., and the Reverend Dr. Victor Rogers for their kind advice offered during their review and discussion of earlier versions of this chapter.

1. M. G. Bloche, "Physician, Turn Thyself In," *New York Times*, June 10, 2004, p. 27; L. S. Rubenstein "Stop Torture: Independent Investigation Needed for Abu Ghraib Crisis," *Physicians for Human Rights Record* 17 (2004): 1, 6.

2. Rubenstein, "Stop Torture"; P. Slevin and J. Stephens, "Detainees' Medical Records Shared," *Hartford Courant*, June 10, 2004, p. A11.

3. R. J. Lifton, "Doctors and Torture," *New England Journal of Medicine* 351 (2004): 415–16.

4. E. E. H. Griffith, "Personal Storytelling and the Metaphor of Belonging," *Diversity and Mental Health* 1 (1995): 29–37.

5. R. Wright, *Native Son* (New York: Perennial Classics, 1991).

6. D. J. Levinson et al., *Seasons of a Man's Life* (New York: Alfred A. Knopf, 1978).

7. H. L. Gates Jr., *Thirteen Ways of Looking at a Black Man* (New York: Random House, 1997), xiv.

8. S. Souljah, *No Disrespect* (New York: Times Books, 1994), xiv.

9. E. E. H. Griffith, *Race and Excellence: My Dialogue with Chester Pierce* (Iowa City: University of Iowa Press, 1998).

10. Gates, *Thirteen Ways*.

11. W. E. Cross Jr., *Shades of Black: Diversity in African-American Identity* (Philadelphia: Temple University Press, 1991).

12. H. L. Gates Jr., *Colored People* (New York: Vintage Books, 1995), xiii.

13. Ibid., xiv.

14. Ibid., xv.

15. See, e.g., R. Kennedy, *Race, Crime, and the Law* (New York: Pantheon Books, 1997); H. O. P. Freeman and R. Payne, "Racial Injustice in Health Care," *New England Journal of Medicine* 342 (2000): 1045–47; H. J. Geiger, "Race and Health Care: An American Dilemma," *New England Journal of Medicine* 335 (1996): 815–16.

16. L. Brent, *Incidents in the Life of a Slave Girl* (New York: Harcourt Brace Jovanovich, 1973).

17. D. Lithwick, "Another Side of Clarence Thomas," *New York Times Book Review*, September 5, 2004, p. 10.

18. S. Lawrence-Lightfoot, *I've Known Rivers: Lives of Loss and Liberation* (New York: Addison-Wesley, 1994), 10.

19. A. L. Higginbothan Jr., "Justice Clarence Thomas in Retrospect," *Hastings Law Journal* 45 (1994): 1405–33.

20. T. A. Parham, "Cycles of Psychological Nigrescence," *Counseling Psychologist* 17 (1989): 187–226.

21. E. E. H. Griffith, "An Open Letter to Black Medical Students: On Belonging at Yale," *Yale Psychiatric Quarterly* 13 (1990): 3–4, 13–15.

22. H. E. Flack and E. D. Pellegrino, *African-American Perspectives on Biomedical Ethics* (Washington, DC: Georgetown University Press, 1992).

23. Griffith, *Race and Excellence*.

24. Lawrence-Lightfoot, *I've Known Rivers*.

25. Cross, *Shades of Black*.

26. Parham, "Cycles of Psychological Nigrescence."

27. Gates, *Thirteen Ways*, xviii.

28. Flack and Pellegrino, *African-American Perspectives*.

29. E. E. Sampson, "Identity Politics: Challenges to Psychology's Understanding," *American Psychologist* 48 (1993): 1219–30.

30. A. A. Stone, "The Ethics of Forensic Psychiatry: A View from the Ivory Tower," in *Law, Psychiatry, and Morality* (Washington, DC: American Psychiatric Press, 1984), 57–75, at 65.

31. Ibid., 68.

32. P. S. Appelbaum, "A Theory of Ethics for Forensic Psychiatry," *Journal of the American Academy of Psychiatry and the Law* 25 (1997): 233–47, at 238.

33. Ibid.
34. E. E. H. Griffith, "Ethics in Forensic Psychiatry: A Cultural Response to Stone and Appelbaum," *Journal of the American Academy of Psychiatry and the Law* 26 (1998): 171–84.
35. P. C. Davis, "Law as Microaggression," *Yale Law Journal* 98 (1989): 1559–77; P. Butler, "Racially Based Jury Nullification: Black Power in the Criminal Justice System," *Yale Law Journal* 105 (1995): 677–725.
36. P. J. Candilis, R. Martinez, and C. Dording, "Principles and Narrative in Forensic Psychiatry: Toward a Robust View of Professional Role," *Journal of the American Academy of Psychiatry and the Law* 29 (2001): 167–73.
37. Cross, *Shades of Black*.

CHAPTER 7

Does an African American Perspective Alter Clinical Ethical Decision Making at the Bedside?

Reginald L. Peniston

THE QUESTION in the title of this chapter is just the type of query for which Friedrich Nietzsche would have had scathing commentary. He might have asked, "Does a German, or Christian, or European perspective alter clinical ethical decision making at the bedside?" He would likely say, "Yes, and in a frightening and self-conscious fashion." Any perspective tied to group thinking would be an artifice of meaningful ethics. I believe that Nietzsche did engage in a bit of sleight-of-hand when judging motives by outcomes and incentives; however his skepticism and condescension are not traits alien to physicians. My first chief of surgery reportedly said, "You can teach any monkey to operate—surgical judgment is the hard part." As a surgeon, jealously respectful of philosophers, I regard philosophical reflection as harder still to teach. Bioethicists, especially those who are physicians or physician extenders, reflect on moral issues complicating all aspects of modern health care. I posit that healing processes and encounters exist prior to the realization of a dilemma or moral conflict. The salutary good of biomedicine precedes the angst of moral doubts. The healing arts become refined as a reaction to and reflection of our injury, our insanity, or our corporal corruption. I refer to biomedicine because science and technology have totally and completely eclipsed the good intentions of those who would heal by magic. This is not to say that when desperate patients resort to faith healers, that if it be for minor complaints or hopeless situations, they will not indeed improve.

As I attempt a response—not necessarily an answer—to the question that frames this chapter, let me reveal a guarded opinion, a further bias I have regarding the exercise of such problems. Clinical ethics as commented on by clinicians, professional clinical ethicists, various hospital ethics committees, and professional organizations has not always maintained proximity to academic bioethics and its various commentators and thinkers. Bioethicists, some of whom are in the news, have the uneasy task of wading through and explaining the difficulties of applied ethics, often without the support of that branch of academic philosophy that investigates ethics writ large. Nursing organizations, focus groups, theologians, and other religious representatives and their followers have an even more awkward predicament, because many of them (particularly in the West) make claims to the elements of caring, feeling, compassion, and even healing that biomedicine with all of its scientific and technological tools has made available. Attempts to introduce difficult metaphysical concepts such as spirituality into the curriculum and the research agenda must be the result of their disillusion with medical technologies and physician and research motives. Indeed, promoting improved access to healing technology, whether in public health or tertiary care, represents the single biggest failure of expert panels of bioethicists—partly because such institutions do not give priority to exploring relevant health care policy, something controlled by governments and political machines. From the outset we know that injustices perpetrated against our largest minority group (the poor and near poor) is a national embarrassment.

Unbridled American materialism continues to cloak itself in the sanctity of marketplace dynamics as uniquely suited to human fulfillment. Indeed, even nature is portrayed as a divinely ordained lottery or marketplace. It is played out in a hierarchy of genetic or racial endowment. Celebrating diversity is not a real antidote to the happenstance of natural inferiority. Confusion as to the good confronts us in the very nature of biological diversity. There is a spontaneous "bad" or "abnormal" in nature—thus confusion as to man's purposeful ends. Those beautiful yet frightening Hubble deep space photographs of worlds ending and beginning give us pause as to the evanescence of our existence as a species or as a permanent part of the universe. Does the universe need us to survive? Perhaps our gods need something like us for company or to add meaning to their existence. But back to the question: Is there a distinctive African American bioethics? Most of what has ever been stated on that subject has left me skeptical, including some of Jorge Garcia's commentary on the matter about a decade ago. I will risk the prediction that Dr. Garcia has not defined that perspective in the manner that follows. And if he has, well, perhaps there will be a little less embarrassment for me.

If I am, by definition, an African American, is my perspective representative or only one of many possible African American perspectives? Is perspective biologically determined, culturally determined, influenced by intelligence quotients or by gender? If one claims to have a Jewish perspective, is it based on the totality of Jewish cultural and historical life? Does it mean that I perseverate on the Holocaust? Depending on the subject, the various factions of Judaism have remarkably different opinions. Where dogmatic beliefs hold sway over freedom of thought (the condition of most ideologues), there can certainly be a monolithic and monotonous drone of unity. Do we as African Americans see every event through a prism of color prejudice or a notion of what slavery was like?

The most provocative stimulus to a unique African American perspective, at least in American society, is the ongoing, pervasive, culturally dominant practice of color-based prejudice and injustice. The darker you are, the more arbitrary and repetitive the injustice—not only by the person in the street but by many public servants, leaders in industry, professionals, and the marketplace at large. When combined with other phenotypic characteristics such as musculature, body habitus, facial features, hair characteristics, and so on, the daily insults, slights, denials, and disenfranchisements take on monumental proportions. This is not to negate the strides that younger generations of Americans have made in suppressing negative responses to dark skin and media distortion.

In dramatic fashion, we have seen a broad-based approval and support for darker skinned people such as Colin Powell and Condoleezza Rice, who openly endorse more conservative American values. The eagerness and regime loyalty with which these two supported the American invasion of Iraq have made them indistinguishable from Donald Rumsfeld, Paul Wolfowitz, Dick Cheney, and George W. Bush. Their decisions may have spelled doom for many thousands of innocent Iraqi citizens and a growing number of American soldiers, but I suspect that many professional politicians and citizens at large take pride in knowing that at least certain African American perspectives have finally come of age. In the case of Colin Powell, the professional soldier seemed unhesitating in following orders. The statesman in him may have reluctantly pursued this problematic and aggressive course, but his criticisms remained muted at best.

Whether Powell and Rice have put forward an opinion that represents a significant portion of the African American population is unknown to me. I recently had a conversation with a close female relative who admitted that she felt that many, if not most, whites held a contemptuous view of dark-skinned peoples. She based this opinion in part on the numerous conversations she overheard by white women in particular—usually in bathrooms and lounges—where because of her light skin she was not identified as an African American. Unlike me, she felt that the invasion of Iraq was prudent and necessary. Because she is married to a Baptist minister who pastors an overwhelmingly black congregation, I inquired as to views among other church members. They were overwhelmingly against this war. In contrast to her experience, I have found prejudicial remarks concerning African Americans to be few and far between when in the company of white physicians who do not know me. From my perspective, the average physician is more comfortable with racial or ethnic diversity and morally superior to the average citizen in that regard. This is as it should be.

We might ask, "Who exemplifies an African American perspective in politics, Al Sharpton or Alan Keyes?" Both men have chosen to be active politicians and both display social advocacy for our citizens at large. If they were physicians, would their approach to biomedical ethics have some nuance dictated by the ill-defined "African American perspective"? It is more likely that their personal philosophies would be decisive. Would they differ in those political decisions and attempts at consensus building, which brings us in line with other industrial societies in guaranteeing access to health care and removing health care from the ruthlessness of the marketplace? I believe the answer is a qualified yes. If they were surgeons, would their previous exposure to color prejudice or other perceptions important to an African American perspective give them a particular insight or expertise regarding thorny clinical dilemmas? I believe the answer is a qualified no.

In the aftermath of the Cold War, pride and arrogance have accompanied all things American. Manipulating the fear and fury subsequent to the September 11, 2001, attacks, and realizing our position of elite military and economic dominance, have further invited notions of American moral superiority by conservatives everywhere. Even ethnic diversity can now be celebrated by the right, as long as it promotes American hegemony and aspirations to Empire. In *The Right Nation*, Micklethwaite and Wooldridge describe this worshiping of America:

American conservatives have an almost sacramental conception of their country. They regard it as a "promised land," a "sanctuary on earth for individual man," "the last best hope of man on earth." And, of course, "a city on a hill." For American conservatives, America is not just a geographical reality; it is the material expression of a spiritual ideal. Ronald Reagan was perhaps the most articulate exponent of this elemental conservative belief. He believed that God had chosen America as the agent of His special purpose on earth. Because America embodied the Democratic ideal, because it hopes to bring that ideal to the rest of the world, it was not condemned to decay, in the way that the Roman and British Empire's had decayed.[1]

In health care, this zealous allegiance is expressed as a constant reference to our superior technology, the best medicine in the world and the "emperor has no clothes" type delusion about the fate of the uninsured. We have little to learn from other societies, in this or any other regard. The human condition abroad may be a legitimate concern, but only the particulars of democratic society, epitomized and sanctified by the dogma of our Constitution (especially as interpreted by the original intent of our gifted founding fathers) addresses that condition in an ethically proper way. The healing arts in other societies, especially socialized medicine abroad, deserves our contempt. Herbert Marcuse predicted the repression of free and creatively wholesome human thought by the harsh and narrow ideologies present in advanced industrial societies some forty years ago.

One-dimensional thought is systematically promoted by the makers of politics and their purveyors of mass information. Their universe of discourse is populated by self-validating hypotheses, which, incessantly and monopolistically repeated, become hypnotic definitions or dictations. For example, "free" are the institutions which operate (and are operated on) in the countries of the Free World; other transcending modes of freedom, are by definition, either anarchism, communism, or propaganda. "Socialistic" are all encroachments on private enterprises not undertaken by private enterprise itself (or by government contracts), such as universal and comprehensive health insurance, or the protection of nature from all too sweeping commercialization, or the establishment of public services, which may hurt private profit. This totalitarian logic of accomplished facts has its Eastern counterpart. There, freedom is the way of life instituted by a Communist régime, and all other transcending modes of freedom are either capitalistic, or revisionist, or leftist sectarianism. In both camps, non-operational ideas are non-behavioral and subversive. The movement of thought is stopped at barriers which appear as the limits of Reason itself.[2]

Canada is formally a capitalist society and has a fee-for-service health care system. The fact that it is a single-payer system with provincial governments serving as fiduciary agents has led to the resentment and distortions promoted by American health insurers, health care institutions, and private providers, who fear alleged decreased quality of care, limited options, and a loss of personal income with any similar health care reforms in the United States. Other than the group known as Physicians for a National Health Plan, there is no staunch support for a Canadian-style system in this country. Although the National Medical Association stood alone in supporting the Medicare legislation of the 1960s, it has since remained firmly in the conservative ranks of private practitioners. The particulars of an American (or African American) liberal or conservative democratic perspective are insufficient to augment or diminish the universal human good promoted by the healing arts. The good that medicine accomplishes is not diminished by the ethnic identity of patients or health care providers or political affiliations. It is not diminished by a particular religious conviction (or lack thereof). It is generally superior in any head-to-head competition with a false god. It is not diminished by geographical location. It is not diminished by who pays the bill. It is not diminished if it is free. In the wrong hands, it can certainly impoverish individuals. It is not intended to get individuals to the other side, although it sometimes speeds the journey. There are those who would extend its impact and nobility well beyond *Homo sapiens* when considering the biosphere in general.

Herbert Marcuse's description of one-dimensional thought as an impediment to reason and therefore reasonableness, and consequently rationality, brings me to the gifted and sober thought of William Augustus Banner. His participation in the symposium on this same subject, fifteen years ago, remains with me today. It has helped me to reflect clearly on the good that is possible in human affairs.

Professor Banner learned ancient and continental philosophy the old-fashioned way: he translated it. Citizenship was profoundly meaningful to him. In *Moral Norms and Moral Order: The Philosophy of Human Affairs*, he wrote:

> Law is the common authority of free individuals who, in their role as citizens, impose upon themselves that order, which is both ex-pressive and protective of their freedom. Law in its very idea as ra-tional governments expresses what is just and fair. Law simply pub-lishes and enforces what morality requires. . . . Justice itself stands forth as a moral norm. To be observed evenly in the law, whether in the correction of wrongdoing or the distribution of goods and services, in the protection of civil liberties or the preservation of safety and peace.[3]

If there is a true and recognizable African American perspective, it cer-tainly and fundamentally includes a concern for justice, and its frequent de-nial to people of color. The frequent disconnect and differentiation between the ethical and the legal by medical ethicists may have contributed to our national failure to adopt policies of universal health access. Where the law is silent, the marketplace finds a home. Many have speculated that denying care to the poor or underinsured is a circuitous proxy for antiminority sentiments.

The good that we seek to achieve in biomedicine is a conscious deci-sion on the part of those who pursue the healing arts. But the practical good inherent in this enterprise requires only a belief in the value of human life here and now. The metaphysical leap to life everlasting or divine nothingness is neither necessary nor sufficient. The same holds for other important needs, desires, and motives. The deliberateness with which we pursue the medical enterprise places it squarely within Banner's description of a ratio-nal, moral order.

> Distinct societies can be thought of as carrying forward, under similar or different conditions, the same general program, of hu-man good, such that an individual's well-being in one society would not differ substantially from another individual's well-being in another society.

The idea of one rational moral order is really entailed in any recognition of a norm distinguishable from the preference of feeling or taste. What is discernible as fair, for example, holds for all persons or for all persons in similar situations. Within the broad unity of one moral order there would obtain, of course, that diversity in practice, that would be required in meeting the precise needs of individuals and groups under the variable conditions of human existence. There is indeed, a richness and significance in the practices that are arrangements or orderings appropriate to different situations. Historical and anthropological accounts provide, in this connection, materials for reflection on the adequacy or suitability of patterns of behavior or modes of life viewed as arising from rational choice and not from biological (racial) or geographical determination.

The rational moral order, embracing both uniformity, and diversity of practice, can be thought to be realizable as an alternative to any and all orders that are parochial in character and foundation. In every parochial order, there is confusion between universality and particularity. A parochial order is one in which the interests of particular individuals or particular groups (ethnic, economic, political, religious) become expressed in terms of the common good and thus take on the guise and sanction of universality. There is the sharpest contrast between the social posture in which particular ends (and means) fall under and are governed by universal ends and the posture in which particular and partisan ends are put forth as having the character and validity of the universal. The rational moral order is simply the system of life, resting upon universal or common claims, which, *as rights*, determine the range of social policy and the range of corresponding duties.

To talk of rights in a responsible and instructive way is to take on a difficult task in the present-day confusion about the just claims of the individual in society. . . . If one comes to believe, with Bentham that a right without the power adequate to its exercise is really a nonentity, a mere philosophical fiction, it is but a short step to believe that "adequate power" is the real ground of right in society and to contend that the advancement of rights is at bottom the pretension of those who have or who seek the resources to promote their own interests and to prevail over others.[4]

Surprisingly, even Banner cannot resist the temptation to give some credibility or credence to a notion of biological or racial determinism. Certainly, he would see its manipulation, as a parochial interest. A more typical parochial interest would be convincing voters that a move to socialized medicine means a loss of personal choice in selecting a physician, a violation of their personal rights, and a decrement in the quality and quantity of their health care. Organized medicine (physicians and insurers) revisits the notion that justice before the law is a manipulated tool of the politically well connected and powerful—a cynical view that Plato considered but disputed. Although we have tremendous difficulties with resource allocation and meeting the increased patient population with a safety net, the Veterans Health Administration has received particular notice from the Institute of Medicine for its quality of care and its patient monitoring techniques.

At the Bedside

Does an African American perspective alter clinical ethical decision making at the bedside? I know of no studies or even any anecdotal reports to suggest an answer. I can say that, after seeing African American physicians treat a diverse population of patients, the more usual traits of personality and professional competence reveal the usual spectrum of bedside manner and adherence to ethical standards and professional etiquette.

Given the still very small percentage of African Americans in the healing arts, it would be very difficult to quantify some amount of African American perspective with which to rank practitioners, and it would be difficult to tabulate some range of ethical clinical issues. While on the faculty of Howard University College of Medicine I did suggest to the medical director of the Howard University Hospital (HUH) that it would be interesting to publish our experience with rates and types of risk management cases and malpractice litigations, as we had a clinical faculty and medical staff that was overwhelmingly minority and a patient population that remained 97 percent black since 1900. Although the mix of payors revealed a much higher proportion of self-pay and Medicaid patients at HUH, the majority of payors were still private insurance carriers. I naively thought this would make an interesting comparison to predominately white hospitals. I was refused emphatically and completely. I admit that an analysis of medical lawsuits or risk management cases obtains no obvious connection to legitimate ethical issues, although some overlap is probable.

I would venture to guess that most African American physicians, not unlike many female physicians, have anecdotes about conflicts with patients or colleagues who are sexist or racist. This leads into a very different area of dealing with individual and institutional injustices. When physicians are confronted with patients who express hostility regarding the ethnic background of their providers—these are clearly mundane matters that are simply resolved. Still, it would seem reasonable to assume, in those clinical, ethical issues marked by concerns for justice, that African American physicians and other African American health care workers would show greater sensitivity.

Notes

The views expressed in this chapter are those of the author and do not represent the views of the Department of Veterans Affairs.

1. John Micklethwait and Adrian Wooldridge, *The Right Nation: Conservative Power in America* (New York: Penguin Press, 2004), 342–43.
2. Herbert Marcuse, *One-Dimensional Man*, 2nd ed. (Boston: Beacon Press, 1991), 14.
3. William A. Banner, *Moral Norms and Moral Order: The Philosophy of Human Affairs* (Gainesville: University Press of Florida, 1981), 101.
4. Ibid., 97–98.

CHAPTER 8

Race, Genetics, and Ethics

Kevin FitzGerald and Charmaine Royal

ON AUGUST 24, 2004, *Boston Globe* correspondent Carolyn Johnson reported on a controversial development in the study of a new combination of drugs (BiDil) for heart failure. The controversy arose because the African American Heart Failure Trial (A-HeFT), the clinical trial for BiDil, sponsored by NitroMed, was halted prematurely after it was found to significantly extend the lives of African Americans who have had heart failure. The results of the study, subsequently published in the *New England Journal of Medicine* (*NEJM*) were in contrast to earlier results that showed no significant benefit for white patients.[1] The reporter summed up the situation: "So, if the government doesn't approve BiDil, it would deny African-Americans treatment for a disease that strikes them earlier than whites, often with a deadly outcome; if it does approve it, some will accuse the government of racism and bad science."[2]

This controversy surrounding the use of racial categories in health care is by no means limited to the BiDil trial. Many times in the past several years this controversy has made national headlines as research has been interpreted to indicate that there are genetic differences among groups that have traditionally been labeled as separate races.[3] In fact, connections between this current research and early twentieth-century eugenics claims are often drawn when such research gains national attention.[4] Because the research into the genetic differences among individuals and groups is not likely to slow down anytime soon, due to the much-touted promise of genomic medicine, various stakeholders have taken clear positions on the possible connections between genetic differences and racial categories. With its own large investment in the Human Genome Project (HGP) and its contributions to genomic medicine, the Department of Energy (DOE) Office of Science states succinctly on its website: "Studies of human variations have determined that there is no scientific basis for race and that 'races' cannot be distinguished genetically.[5]

If this statement is accurate, why is there still interest in using racial categories along with genetic information in medical research and clinical care, and should there be such interest? As one may suspect, the answers to this question—like the concepts of race, health, and genetic constitution—are not simple or easily delineated. However, due to the history of racial conflict and eugenics in this country, these answers are extremely important in helping to frame a more ethical and just approach to bringing the benefits of genomic medicine to everyone in need.

We will address the issue of race, genomic medicine, and ethics in three parts. First, we explore the concept of "race" and its interface with genomics. Second, we analyze this relationship between race and genomics and its deeper genomic medicine ramifications. Finally, we examine health care and medical research in order to see how one might approach this issue without exacerbating the current disparities in health care or sacrificing the benefits of genomic medicine that can be shared by all.

Race and Genomics

Since the HGP revealed that, on average, any two unrelated persons share over 99.9 percent of their DNA sequences,[6] the relationship between race and genomics has increasingly become the focus of investigations and discussions.[7] In a recent article titled "Deconstructing the Relationship between Genetics and Race," the authors contend that the current controversy surrounding the use of racial categories "has been fostered by the conflation of several issues." These issues include "whether individuals can be reliably allocated into valid genetic clusters in which all members share more recent common ancestry than members of other clusters, whether descriptors such as race or ethnicity capture any of the genetic differences between such clusters, and whether these differences are meaningful for health-related variation among groups."[8]

Though some current research strongly indicates that genetic data can help distinguish individuals in various groups from one another, the authors of this article conclude that racial categories are, at best, quite limited in their usefulness in medical research, especially when correlated with genetic information.[9] They bolster their conclusion by distinguishing between biogeographical ancestry and race. It may well be that genetic foundations for disease risk will sort according to proportions of one's individual ancestries—presuming, of course, that these proportions can be made clear. However, biogeographical ancestry does not necessarily correlate well with social conceptions of race, especially when the concepts are applied across societal and cultural boundaries.[10]

The preceding observations have been further corroborated more recently by scientists in the September 2004 *Nature Genetics* supplement titled "Genetics for the Human Race." The supplement, supported in part by the DOE and the National Human Genome Research Institute (NHGRI), primary funders of the HGP, arguably provided a comprehensive examination of the "state of the science on human genome variation and 'race.' " The contributors generally agree that genetic variation, though exhibiting some correlations with traditional concepts of "race," is distributed in a continuous and overlapping pattern across populations and is geographically structured according to historical patterns of genetic drift, gene flow, mutation, migration, and natural selection.[11] They also agree that traditionally defined "races" are not homogenous groups and that the observed correlations with genetic variation and health outcomes are imprecise and reflective of various surrogate relationships.[12]

There appears to be less congruence among the authors, however, with regard to the appropriate steps for moving forward in light of the current scientific evidence. All authors acknowledge the inadequacy and imperfection of "race" as a proxy for various genetic and nongenetic factors and call for better-designed and more inclusive investigations to delineate more concrete variables that influence health and response to treatment. However, some believe that despite its limitations, "race" is a useful health-related variable that should not be disregarded in research and health care.[13] Mountain and Risch further suggest that "racial" or "ethnic" categories serve as valuable predictors of health outcomes and should continue to be used in epidemiological research, at least until more appropriate descriptors or correlates have been identified.[14] Others,[15] like Bamshad and colleagues,[16] maintain that ancestry (not "race") provides a more accurate and useful measure of genetic variation and its relationship to health.

In addition, Keita and colleagues of African descent investigating genetic and environmental contributors to diseases common in African Americans and other African Diaspora populations challenge the very use of the term *race* in its application to humans.[17] They contend that given the preponderance of scientific data indicating that the human species does not structure into homogenous, discontinuous units, no divisions of humans (including the standard anthropological "racial" classifications) meet the kinds of divergence criteria outlined by Avise and Ball that would justify calling them races (or subspecies).[18] Of particular relevance to this discussion of African American perspectives on biomedical ethics is the pronouncement of Kieta and colleagues that the U.S. census groups are not races, but are sociodemographic groups, exhibiting biogeographical, biological (including genetic), sociohistorical, and cultural variation within and among them, that must be factored into health-related investigations.

Kieta and colleagues hasten to emphasize that the nonexistence of human races does not translate into the nonexistence of racism (defined as the systematic oppression of groups deemed to be "fundamentally biologically different"), which they point out must be addressed. For these researchers, it is not acceptable to state that "there is no biological basis for race" in humans, yet continue to use the terms *race* and *racial* in describing human groups. Maintaining the concept of race for humans does imply that the groups traditionally indicated as such are true races, and this unique contradiction between scientific findings and the application of those findings may actually be the primary source of the scientific and social conundrum that we currently face regarding the issue of "race."

Keita and colleagues advocate not for cessation in conducting population studies or labeling participating groups, but instead for linguistic precision, using terms that are based on known scientific and other evidence, in describing human populations. In addition, they encourage researchers to avoid "generalizations that invoke 'genetic' explanations," utilizing more careful and accurate descriptions of demographic groups under study.

Do these conclusions mean that those who argue for the use of racial categories in medical research are completely in error? Some may say not necessarily, because as indicated by Bamshad and colleagues, some correlations of race with political and socioeconomic factors might be useful, particularly with regard to environmental effects on the health of particular individuals and groups.[19] Conversely, others such as Keita et al. (2004) will likely respond, yes—and no.[20] Yes, if by saying "racial" they are, based on the established definition of the word, implying natural and inherent evolutionary distinctions; no, if they are referring to sociodemographic categories or groups, in which case, they should state it as such—"sociodemographic." As acknowledged by Keita and colleagues, "Terms and labels have qualitative implications." The labeling of groups may be inevitable or even necessary in biomedical (including genomic) research and practice, but it needs to be done with greater precision.

Genomic medicine has shown much promise. If sociodemographic categories prove useful for genomic research and medicine, then those who argue for the abolition of these categories due to their history of abuse would face an even more difficult struggle.

Race and Genomic Medicine

The current and potential impacts of the HGP on the practice of medicine are, without question, revolutionary.[21] In describing findings related to human genome variation, Guttmacher and Collins declared that

> except for monozygotic twins, each person's genome is unique. All physicians will soon need to understand the concept of genetic variability, its interactions with the environment, and its implications for patient care. With the sequencing of the human genome, the practice of medicine has now entered an era in which the individual patient's genome will help determine the optimal approach to care, whether it is preventive, diagnostic, or therapeutic. Genomics, which has quickly emerged as the central basic science of biomedical research, is poised to take center stage in clinical medicine as well.[22]

How much attention is given currently to the promise of genomic medicine? One indication of its significance is a collection of articles in the September 2004 edition of *Nature Review Genetics*. These articles focus on one of the most discussed areas of genomic medicine: pharmacogenetics/genomics. In reviewing how genetic information might impact our treatment of disease with drugs, Urs Meyer states, "The future impact of [pharmacogenetics] and pharmacogenomics is likely to be considerable both in the selection of the right drug at the proper 'individual' dose and in the prevention of adverse effects. By translating the increasing knowledge of human genetic diversity into better drug treatment, improved health through personalized therapy remains a realistic future scenario in many fields of medicine."[23]

This "realistic future" also raises some concerns. While individualized or personalized medicine is an anticipated outcome of genomic medicine, we are not there yet, at least not on a large scale. Consequently, and perhaps naturally, this interim period increasingly fosters the need to study group variation in health and response to therapeutics. In a companion article, several health care experts warn of the problems that pharmacogenetics/genomics might bring. Alasdair Breckenridge mentions that "this approach does run the risk of increasing the complexity of health-care delivery and perhaps of exacerbating existing inequalities in health-care delivery."[24] More specifically addressing the inequalities, Helen Wallace states, "Poorer populations might be excluded from drug testing altogether, and racism and inequalities could be exacerbated."[25] And Mark Rothstein concludes, "There might be considerable social costs in stratifying society into genotype-matched groups for the purposes of pharmaceutical development and marketing, especially when some polymorphisms of pharmaceutical significance might be correlated to varying degrees with groups categorized by race or ethnicity."[26] In contrast to these predictions, Klaus Lindpaintner argues:

The specific issue raised by some—namely that PGx [pharmacogenetics] will be used to substitute for racial discrimination and will lead to discrimination against the emerging economies—would appear to be unsupported by any evidence. First, the medical deprivation of the Southern hemisphere is fundamentally a problem of North–South mal-distribution of wealth. However, it should be noted that the pharmaceutical industry has demonstrated a commitment to supply certain drugs that are approved in industrialized nations at greatly reduced costs to emerging economies to meet local medical needs. Second, 95% of genetic variation is within-(ethnic/racial) group and 5% is between-group—so there is no rationale to use genetics as a substitute for "race" (a multifactorial concept that is viewed today as rooted far more in socio-

economics than in biology). Third, if anything, using a more specific test than skin colour with regard to likely response to a treatment will allow the replacement of racial stereotypes, rather than
their enhancement.[27]

This apparent disagreement between Lindpaintner and the other authors may be due more to a difference in perspective than in substance. Lindpaintner is emphasizing how people might rationally or logically respond
to the information gleaned from genetic research when applying it to our
current health care situations. Though his data may be accurate, one could
easily argue that societies and nations may not follow his predicted course in
their interpretation and use of genetic research and information. In fact, due
to the complexities of social and political structures throughout the world,
the very nature of the information gleaned from genetic research could actually result in all the above prognostications coming true at the same time.

Regardless of whose prediction concerning the impact of pharmaco-
genetics/genomics comes true, the statements of the authors cited earlier
indicate the importance of the issue of race and genomic medicine. Even if
research shows no link between sociodemographic categories and genetic
foundations of disease, the current reality of health care disparities among
minority communities means that any advances in genomic medicine might
exacerbate this disparity. In the past several years, a variety of extensive investigations have clarified a pervasive problem facing health care efforts in
the United States—severe disparities in health and health care among various racial and ethnic communities. As an Institute of Medicine (IOM) report states: "Disparities in health care are among this nation's most serious
health care problems. Research has extensively documented the pervasive-
ness of racial and ethnic disparities."[28] If the advances in health care research
and technology have led us to this tragic situation, then we must look seriously at how advances in genomic medicine might need to be pursued and
employed in order to, at the very least, not exacerbate this tragedy.

If human genetic variation is understood to be overlapping and continuous across ethno-ancestral and sociodemographic groups, interacting at
differing frequencies with various cultural, social, psychological, and other
environmental factors to influence health and treatment outcomes, then reliance on group membership as the sole (or even the primary) criterion for
determination of health status and health care is questionable. The existing
disparities in health care are indeed symptomatic of flawed scientific think-

ing (or misapplication of scientific data) in the context of an already in-equitable social system—a system that pervasively marginalizes socio-demographic groups deemed to be inferior. Therefore, in order for genomic medicine to proceed in ways that could abate and not exacerbate health care disparities, the scientific community must be a catalyst for social change. That is to say, the scientific community must illuminate the fact that the true nature and biology of human relationships is a factor in dissecting the construct of health and disease.

With regard to pharmacogenomics, the need to move beyond macro-designations to more precise descriptions of groups is critical to increasing understanding of the biological and environmental mechanisms of action of medicines, thereby optimizing delineation of the target group and mini-mizing injustice. The case of BiDil serves as a timely example. Given the historical experiences of African Americans in the United States, the announcement regarding BiDil was perceived by many African Americans as a welcome change in that biomedical research finally generated a product specifically designed to help "blacks."[29] However, it may be appropriate to ask some critical questions, such as, "Who were the 'African Americans' in the study?" "What were their biological, cultural, and geographic backgrounds?" In light of the range of genetic and environmental heterogeneity within the "African American" or "black American" population, as well as our knowledge of populations in general, it is inevitable that BiDil will not benefit all African Americans with heart failure and will be effective for some persons from other populations. If approved by the FDA as a drug for "African Americans," how will BiDil be dispensed in the clinical setting? What will be the inclusion and exclusion criteria for dispensation? Will effective treatments be sought for African Americans who do not respond positively to BiDil? Will members of other populations for whom BiDil may be effective have equal access to the drug?

These are only a few of the types of questions that should guide regulatory decisions regarding the approval of "group-specific" medicines. It is important to note, however, that the development of "ethnic" drugs by pharmaceutical companies is initially driven by numerous factors, not the least of which is economics.[30] Bloche suggested that the intellectual property protection held by NitroMed would likely not have been extended by thirteen years if the drug had been promoted as a treatment for all heart failure patients, regardless of ethno-ancestry. He further pointed out that market and regulatory incentives shape research agendas, in that "the ease with which

race can be used as a crude marker for clinically relevant biologic difference makes it attractive as a basis for bringing pharmaceutical products to market."[31] Even more disconcerting is the reality that patent protection for and regulatory approval of such products serve as disincentives for the pharmaceutical companies involved to sponsor research to elucidate mechanisms of action.[32] Taylor and colleagues, the A-HeFT investigators, acknowledged the need for future research "to identify genotypic and phenotypic characteristics that would transcend racial or ethnic categories to identify a population with heart failure in which there is an increased likelihood of a favorable response to such therapy."[33] It remains to be seen whether NitroMed will actually take the lead in sponsoring efforts that could facilitate equity in health care for heart failure, thereby helping to bridge the gap between science and ethics.

The Future of Health Care

Biomedical research and health care are undeniably linked. The following prognosis for the future of health care in the genomic era is informed by further assessment of various conceptualizations of the relationships among race, genomics, and genomic medicine, and by consideration of the potential scientific, ethical, and social impacts of these conceptualizations on research and medical practice in general.

In the Lindpaintner quotation,[34] there is mention of how genetics cannot rationally be used as a substitute for racial categories, in part because race is viewed as rooted more in socioeconomics than in biology. Considering the socioeconomic correlations between "racial" minorities and health care disparities cited above, one could become even more concerned for the future of health care as a result of Lindpaintner's comments. Some might ask, "Why give BiDil any special consideration if indeed there is no genetic basis for a difference between the African American patients and white patients?" Though the people involved in the BiDil trial, as well as many other health care workers, could easily respond that the nongenetic differences between the two patient groups may well explain both the differences in disease prevalence and therapeutic response, their answer might be drowned out in the growing wave of genomic medicine. In other words, while it is the case that genetic research produces data that contradict any biological support for racial categorization among humans, the growing emphasis on looking for answers to health care issues from genetic research may skew our responses to health care problems and give undue attention and concern to those that can be addressed primarily from a genetic standpoint.

Every day Americans are inundated with reports of the latest discoveries in molecular and genetic research. As we struggle to make health care decisions and policies regarding where to put our confidence, our hope, and hence, our resources, the chorus we hear the most is that this research will be our best bet to solve our health care problems. Considering the evidence that has revealed the growing tragedy of health care disparities within our own country, not to mention the greater disparities worldwide, one can rightly question whether or not this reliance on cutting-edge research is realistic—and for whom? This is not raised as a question of the need for medical research in general. The point is to force us to connect more directly our purported goals in health care and our means. This connection between goals and means helps explain the apparent disconnect between Lindpaintner and the other previously quoted commentators.

The question, ultimately, is not *whether* genomic medicine can be used for good, but rather, *how* it can be used for good. An answer to this question can come only if we know what the good is that we desire. If the good is to develop genomic medicine as a new and powerful option to be placed within our arsenal of therapies and interventions, then the obvious answer would be to go full speed ahead, in line with our current course. However, if the goal is to provide better health care, interpreted broadly to include better lives in general for everyone, then a different approach might be the appropriate answer.

Arguably, improvement in health care in the United States is not likely to occur in the absence of some changes in the conduct and application of science. Much of the research into biological group differences has historically been predicated on the false assumption that "race" appropriately describes human populations, and that the observed differences are innate, immutable, and representative of evolutionary divergence. These assumptions have fostered notions of biological hierarchy, ultimately leading to social hierarchy among human groups. Consequently, science has played a significant role in shaping and maintaining the current inequitable political, economic, educational, and health care systems of our society. The position taken and approach suggested by Keita and colleagues,[35] therefore, might provide a suitable context within which to begin to analyze and address the issue of genomic medicine and health care disparities in the United States.

Given that science has demonstrated that neither the major continental groups nor subgroups within them are races, and because there appears to be general agreement that we should not and perhaps cannot dispense with group labels in biomedical research and clinical care, the challenging question then becomes "What do we do with the term *race*?" As previously mentioned, Keita and others suggest that its use in describing human populations be discontinued and that it be limited to the species for which it is relevant.[36] They further offer alternative terms, such as ethno-ancestry or ethno-ancestral group, that account for the pertinent classification criteria. Others seem comfortable with retaining *race*, and over time, some have redefined this legitimate, already defined biological term to fit the social, legal, and political constructs within which it has been (mis)applied.[37] In light of the obvious confusion with conceptualizing "race" in relation to humans, it may be reasonable to conclude that this is due primarily to the fact that race *is* not appropriate for humans and that the time has probably come to eliminate the term and its ascribed meaning from our vocabulary when describing human groups. However, is this practical? Is it realistic to envision a consistent "no biological race" position for a society as "race"-conscious as the United States? What would this mean for affirmative action and other such programs or endeavors that have been implemented to benefit African Americans and members of other groups that have been marginalized because of pervasive racial thinking? Could this move effect constructive change in our perceptions of ourselves and others? Could it help revolutionize our perspectives on health, disease, and other complex traits in populations and lead to a more just health care system and society?

Indeed, the purging of "race" from the glossary of human attributes is a valid and logical step if current biological evidence is the primary consideration. Undoubtedly, however, there will be broad agreement that such an undertaking and the associated paradigm shift in science, medicine, and society will be formidable at best. Nonetheless, from some ethical perspectives, this purging of "race" could be the most fitting action to address effectively issues of human dignity, beneficence, and justice. Further, the virtue of truth telling arguably requires that we purge "race" from our biological usage. However, it certainly is to the advantage of various political and social agendas for "racial thinking" and perceptions of inherent group differences to persist, thus exacerbating the challenge of integrating accurate and precise genetic information into these and other critical areas of our existence.

It is certainly unrealistic to believe that wishing that "race" had no other connotations will make it so. Still, regardless of what the connotations are or what other definitions have been created, scientists (geneticists in particular) must be the initiators of accurate biological terminology and must conduct science in a way that reflects the reality that humans do not easily subdivide into races. Human genome research is indeed forcing humanity to question and rectify this long-standing misrepresentation of the truth. It is only when scientists operate based on what is known about biological (genetic and other) differences among groups that society can begin to address the plethora of issues that have stemmed from the misapplication of the term *race* to humans. The scientific community does have a unique opportunity and responsibility to positively influence physical as well as social well-being in this regard.

In striving for a more ethical health care system in this genomic era, not only should we reevaluate the use of the term *race*, but we should also exhibit greater care in the use and application of macrodesignations such as African American, European American, and so on. Though valid sociodemographic descriptors, each of these terms often conveys a monolithic identity, thereby compromising the understanding of possible gene-environment effects and impeding the advancement of science, medicine, and society. More detailed investigation and description of populations invariably increases the capacity for the development of more targeted, more equitable, and possibly more effective treatment of disease.

In responding to Carolyn Johnson's commentary,[38] the FDA's decision regarding the approval of BiDil for treatment of heart failure in African Americans must be based on careful consideration of the myriad scientific, ethical, and social implications. It has the potential to revolutionize (for better or for worse) the conduct of science, the practice of medicine, and the future of our society.

Conclusion

Data from genetic research do not support racial categorization of humans. Nonetheless, this information by itself does not guarantee that genetic research and the genomic medicine that comes from it will not add to existing health care disparities among sociodemographic groups. Hence we are faced with an enormous challenge, heightened by the purported promise of genomic medicine, but also applicable to almost every area of medical research and development. The following question continuously arises: If under our current research and health care structures a medical advance is likely to benefit only a relative few, and is likely to exacerbate health care disparities, should we continue to develop and apply this technology in the absence of more critical examination of and greater attention to the root cause(s) of disparities in health and health care?

It is important to clarify that negative answers to this question do not necessarily require that the pursuit of technological advances stop or be abandoned. Negative answers do, however, require a shift in emphasis away from technological solutions to our greatest health care problems to solutions that also incorporate the facets of health and health care not reducible to molecular biology and genetics. The nature and consequence of such a shift could well be a positive answer not only for those who are most in need and most behind in our health care arena but also for the broader U.S. society and humankind as a whole.

Notes

1. A. Taylor et al., "Combination of Isosorbide Dinitrate and Hydralazine in Blacks with Heart Failure," *New England Journal of Medicine* 351, no. 20 (2004): 2049–57.
2. Carolyn Johnson, "Should Medicine Be Colorblind? Debate Erupts over a Drug That Works Better in African-Americans," *Boston Globe*, August 24, 2004, p. C1.
3. R. M. Henig, "The Genome in Black and White (and Gray)," *New York Times Magazine*, October 10, 2004, pp. 47–51.
4. F. D. Roylance, "'A sort of scientific malpractice': Genetics: Scientists Are Cautioning Doctors against the Use of Race as a Guide in Diagnosis, Treatment and Research," *Baltimore Sun*, October 11, 2004, p. A1.
5. DOE, "Human Genome Project Information: Minorities, Race and Genomics" (October 28, 2004). Retrieved October 23, 2006, from www.ornl.gov/hgmis/elsi/minorities.html
6. J. C. Venter et al., "The Sequence of the Human Genome," *Science* 291 (2001): 1304–51.
7. See, e.g., *New England Journal of Medicine* 348 (March 20, 2003): 12. Specific articles include E. G. Phimster, "Medicine and the Racial Divide," pp. 1081–82; R. S. Cooper, J. S. Kaufman, and R. Ward, "Race and Genomics," pp. 1166–70; E. G. Burchard et al., "The Importance of Race and Ethnic Background in Biomedical Research and Clinical Practice," pp. 1170–75.

8. M. Bamshad et al., "Deconstructing the Relationship between Genetics and Race," *Nature Reviews Genetics* 5 (August 2004): 598–609, quote at 598.

9. Ibid., 607–8.

10. Ibid., 607.

11. S. A. Tishkoff and K. K. Kidd, "Implications of Biogeography of Human Populations for 'Race' and Medicine," *Nature Genetics* 36, no. 11 (2004): 21–27; L. B. Jorde and S. P. Wooding, "Genetic Variation, Classification and 'Race,'" *Nature Genetics* 36, no. 11 (2004): 28–33; S. O. Y. Keita et al., "Conceptualizing Human Variation," *Nature Genetics* 36, no. 11 (2004): 17–21; C. N. Rotimi, "Are Medical and Nonmedical Uses of Large-Scale Genomic Markers Conflating Genetics and 'Race'?" *Nature Genetics* 36, no. 11 (2004): 28–33; F. Collins, "What We Do and Don't Know about 'Race,' 'Ethnicity,' Genetics and Health at the Dawn of the Genome Era," *Nature Genetics* 36, no. 11 (2004): 13–15; E. J. Parra, R. A. Kittles, and M. D. Shriver, "Implications of Correlations between Skin Color and Genetic Ancestry for Biomedical Research," *Nature Genetics* 36, no. 11 (2004): 54–59.

12. Tishkoff and Kidd, "Implications"; Jorde and Wooding, "Genetic Variation"; Collins, "What We Do"; M. Cho and P. Sankar, "Forensic Genetics and Ethical, Legal and Social Implications beyond the Clinic," *Nature Genetics* 36, no. 11 (2004): 8–12; C. D. M. Royal and G. M. Dunston, "Changing the Paradigm from 'Race' to Human Genome Variation," *Nature Genetics* 36, no. 11 (2004): 5–7; Keita et al., "Conceptualizing"; J. L. Mountain and N. Risch, "Assessing Genetic Contributions to Phenotype Differences among 'Racial' and 'Ethnic' Groups," *Nature Genetics* 36, no. 11 (2004): S48–S53; Rotimi, "Medical and Nonmedical Uses"; S. K. Tate and D. B. Goldstein, "Will Tomorrow's Medicines Work for Everyone?" *Nature Genetics* 36, no. 11 (2004): 34–42.

13. Collins, "What We Do"; Mountain and Risch, "Assessing Genetic Contributions"; Tate and Goldstein, "Tomorrow's Medicines."

14. Mountain and Risch, "Assessing Genetic Contributions."

15. Tishkoff and Kidd, "Implications"; Jorde and Wooding, "Genetic Variation"; Keita et al., "Conceptualizing."

16. Bamshad et al., "Deconstructing."

17. Keita et al., "Conceptualizing."

18. J. C. Avise and R. M. Ball, "Principles of Genealogical Concordance in Species Concepts and Biological Taxonomy," *Oxford Surveys in Evolutionary Biology* 7 (1990): 45–67.

19. Bamshad et al., "Deconstructing."

20. Keita et al., "Conceptualizing."

21. F. S. Collins et al. "A Vision for the Future of Genomics Research," *Nature* 422 (2003): 835–47; A. Guttmacher and F. S. Collins, "Genomic Medicine: A Primer," *New England Journal of Medicine* 347 (2002): 1512–21.

22. Guttmacher and Collins, "Genomic Medicine," 1520.

23. U. A. Meyer, "Pharmacogenetics: Five Decades of Therapeutic Lessons from Genetic Diversity," *Nature Reviews Genetics* 5 (September 5, 2004): 669–76.

24. A. Breckenridge et al., "Pharmacogenetics: Ethical Problems and Solutions," *Nature Reviews Genetics* 5 (2004): 676–80.

25. Ibid., 678.

26. Ibid., 677.

27. Ibid., 679.

28. Institute of Medicine, "Guidance for the National Healthcare Disparities Report" (Washington, DC: National Academy Press, 2002), 1.

29. C. Page, "Blacks-only Drug Has a Special Place in This Heart," *Chicago Tribune*, November 13, 2004, p. 29.

30. M. G. Bloche, "Race-Based Therapeutics," *New England Journal of Medicine* 351, no. 20 (2004): 2035–37; J. Kahn, "How a Drug Becomes 'Ethnic': Law, Commerce, and the Production of Racial Categories in Medicine," *Yale Journal of Health Policy, Law, and Ethics* 4, no. 1 (2004): 1–46.

31. Bloche, "Race-Based Therapeutics," 2036.

32. Ibid.

33. Taylor et al., "Combination," 2055.

34. Breckenridge et al., "Pharmacogenetics."

35. Keita et al., "Conceptualizing."

36. Ibid.

37. IOM, *Unequal Treatment: Confronting Racial and Ethic Disparities in Health Care* (Washington, DC: National Academy Press, 2003).

38. Johnson, "Should Medicine Be Colorblind?"

AFTERWORD

An African American's Internal Perspective on Biomedical Ethics

Lawrence J. Prograis Jr.

> Most people think that shadows follow, precede or surround beings or objects.
> The truth is that they also surround words, ideas, desires, deeds, impulses
> and memories.
>
> —Elie Wiesel, *The Fifth Son*

Elie Wiesel's articulation of what outlines, casts an illumination, or draws a
rough image not only of objects but also of nonobjects defines a focus on the
context of human life. We all cast shadows within and outside of our lives.
These shadows can be said to be an expression of what defines all humans.
We all arise from some place, some past; we have a context and a history.
We do not rationally reason from within empty vessels. Like shadows, our
perspectives (our perceptions, insights, and beliefs) arise from *within* and
outside us, from our exposure to families, friends, history, religious beliefs,
and our social structures in which we live our lives.[1] It is these places, ideas,
people, and things that bring our present to life and allow us to articulate
topics for the future. Wiesel's theme can be said to resonate from within his
Jewish identity. But what of the perspectives offered within these pages? The
perceptions, beliefs, and insights of African Americans on biomedical
ethics—what do they say and how do they say it? A starting place to explore
these questions is, perhaps, with perception itself.

More than two thousand years ago, Plato in the *Theaetetus* described the position of Protagoras of Abdera in Thrace. "Man is the measure of all things—alike of the being of things that are and of the not-being of things that are not." Thus perception by an individual is the domain of that individual. Plato further understood Protagoras's declaration more specifically, in that he saw perception first to be related to the senses. But he also noted its relationship to moral and aesthetic issues.[2] Today philosophers place these arguments within the domains of "fact and object perception."[3] These are places where the reality of objects and concepts are debated under specific theories. The arguments can get messy and abstract, but one thing is certain: perception, language, conceptual foundations, or scientific theories are defining factors for *interpretation*. As Robert Audi writes, "Seeing facts is much more sensitive (and, hence, relative) to the conceptual resources, the background knowledge and scientific theories, of the observer, and this difference must be kept in mind in evaluating claims about perceptual relativity."[4] One might argue that this is similar to Wiesel's shadows—the shadows (conceptual resources, background knowledge, and scientific theories) that surround our past and present lives, and how we reflect on these objects of reality and ideas. So, if this is true, then Garcia's "standpoint epistemology" and virtue ethics may be a starting point we might all agree upon, that is, we humans may perceive "morally significant features of a situation to which features others are blind."[5]

Bioethics

The Birth of Bioethics, *The Story of Bioethics*, and other texts have been written about the *why, where, who*, and *how* of bioethics in the twentieth century.[6] In the introduction to this book, Edmund Pellegrino writes on the *evolution* of bioethics.[7] Central to all of these histories is the "multidisciplinary" approach brought to bioethics by those involved in its development and by those involved in it today. Beyond the multidisciplinary approach of bioethics, Pellegrino has presented what he sees as a tension between "cultural beliefs about right and good com[ing] into conflict with the more generally promulgated ethical norms of bioethics."[8] He ends with the proverbial question, "Are the normative perspectives of moral philosophy and 'culture' incommensurable, or do they complement and supplement each other?"[9] Albert Jonsen, in *The Birth of Bioethics*, identifies a philosopher, Alasdair MacIntyre, whose interest was in the "social and cultural context of moral argument."[10] Jonsen placed MacIntyre in a class of ethicists who approached ethical analysis from the metaethics point of view.[11] This view, according to Jonsen, was a new approach to moral philosophy. Is it MacIntyre's work and that of others in this realm of philosophical dialogue that may answer Pellegrino's *incommensurable* question?

Within the last decade and a half, such books as *Beyond a Western Bioethics: Voices from the Developing World, Transcultural Dimensions in Medical Ethics, African-American Perspectives on Biomedical Ethics*, and *Bioethics Research Concerns and Directions for African-Americans* have examined the relationship between bioethics and culture.[12] They differ from their more philosophical and anthropological counterparts in that they view moral norms from the particular, that is, within a particular culture, or first person, and from a particular cultural viewpoint. The authors of these books were pioneers who, like MacIntyre, had an interest in the "social and cultural context of moral argument."[13] To this end, what of these individuals who identify themselves as African Americans who reside *within* what has been defined as the African American culture of America?[14]

African American

As we move further into the twenty-first century, genetics and ancestry will be used to further define an individual's scientific *identity*, and the potentially troubling term *race* (a social construct) may move further from the surface of everyday nomenclature or become more generally defined within broader context such as the "human race."[15] For now, we are still faced with the term *race*, and its usage scientifically and socially.

The term *African American*, like other group terms in America, for example, Italian Americans and Irish Americans, is associated with different racial and ethnic groups. These different ancestral identities might be said to be associated with a specific culture. Each individual within these different groups are viewed externally by other individuals and are relegated to a particular group.[16] One's external characteristics as viewed by others and one's *internal perspective* of oneself can either define and embolden identity or produce a conflicting picture of tension between the identifier and the identified. Philosopher Anthony Appiah has written clearly on identity. His notion of identity is a complex mix of liberty, individualism, autonomy, culture, and cosmopolitanism. Appiah notes, "It is also regularly assumed that the tradition is ethically individualist—in the sense that it assumes that, in the end, everything that matters morally, matters because of its impact on individuals—so that if nations, or religious communities, or families matter, they matter because they make a difference to the people who compose them." Appiah thus allows us to view what this writer believes is his *internal perspective* concerning individualism.[17] Space does not permit a full treatment of this notion of *internal perspective*, but it is the hope of this author that the relationship between one's internal perspective and identity should be the topic of further discussions and investigations.

Conclusion

In this Afterword I have sought to bring a different perspective to certain concepts—"bioethics," "African American," and the very term *perspective* itself—which have evoked, and continue to evoke, much dialogue and debate. I have tried to shine a light into the shadows of objects, but also of nonobjects, to better illuminate the internal perspective we all bring to bear on our moral life. It is this internal perspective that should allow J. L. A. Garcia's "standpoint epistemology" to begin a dialogue among the different voices in the field of bioethics—particularly those voices, found in this book, who self-claim the identity of African American.

Notes

The ideas and opinions expressed are the author's views and do not represent any official position or policy of the National Institutes of Health, the Public Health Service, or the Department of Health and Human Services.

1. *The American Heritage Dictionary of the English Language*, 4th ed. (2000) gives the following senses/definitions of perspective: "1a. A view or vista. b. A mental view or outlook: *'It is useful occasionally to look at the past to gain a perspective on the present'* (Fabian Linden). 2. The appearance of objects in depth as perceived by normal binocular vision. 3a. The relationship of aspects of a subject to each other and to a whole: *a perspective of history; a need to view the problem in the proper perspective.* b. Subjective evaluation of relative significance; a point of view: *the perspective of the displaced homemaker.* c. The ability to perceive things in their actual interrelations or comparative importance: *tried to keep my perspective throughout the crisis.* 4. The technique of representing three-dimensional objects and depth relationships on a two-dimensional surface." This broad or general concept tends to connote most of the time a sense of super-

ficial or off-the-cuff reasoning on a particular issue. But another sense of this word is the notion of a deep abiding belief that arises from within and outside of your person. It is this perspective that motivates you, drives you to your actions. An extensive discussion of this concept is for another time, but I suggest its internal elements—perception, *insight*, and belief.

2. Edith Hamilton and Huntington Cairns, *Plato: The Collected Dialogues* (Princeton, NJ: Princeton University Press, 1961).

3. Robert Audi, *The Cambridge Dictionary of Philosophy,* 2nd ed. (Cambridge: Cambridge University Press, 1999), "Perception."

4. Ibid.

5. See Garcia's contribution to this volume, and his discussion of "standpoint epistemology."

6. Jennifer K. Walter and Eran P. Klein, *The Story of Bioethics: From Seminal Works to Contemporary Explorations* (Washington, DC: Georgetown University Press, 2003), and Albert R. Jonsen, *The Birth of Bioethics* (New York: Oxford University Press, 1998).

7. See Pellegrino's introduction to this volume.

8. Ibid.

9. Ibid.

10. Jonsen, *Birth of Bioethics.*

11. Jonsen's (ibid.) articulation here about MacIntyre, in particular his view or metaethical analysis at looking closely on "fragmented moral concepts torn from their cultural roots," lends further clarification and impetus toward the understanding of different conceptual foundations evolving from different cultures.

12. See Angeles T. Alora and Josephine M. Lumitao, *Beyond a Western Bioethics: Voices from the Developing World* (Washington, DC: Georgetown University Press, 2001); Edmund Pellegrino, Pietro Corsi, and Patricia Mazzarella, *Transcultural Dimensions in Medical Ethics* (Frederick, MD: University Publishing Group, 1992); Harley E. Flack and Edmund D. Pellegrino, *African-American Perspectives on Biomedical Ethics* (Washington, DC: Georgetown University Press, 1992); and Marian G. Secundy, Annette Dula, and September Williams, *Bioethics Research Concerns and Directions for African-Americans* (Tuskegee, AL: Tuskegee University National Center for Bioethics in Research and Health Care, Tuskegee Institute, 2000).

13. Jonsen, *Birth of Bioethics.*

14. See a full discussion of "within" by Martin Heidegger, *Being and Time* (San Francisco, CA: Harper San Francisco, 1962).

15. Francis S. Collins, "What We Do and Don't Know about 'Race,' 'Ethnicity,' Genetics and Health at the Dawn of the Genome Era," *Nature Genetics Supplement* 36 (2004): S13–S15.

16. Kwame A. Appiah and Amy Gutmann, *Color Conscious: The Political Morality of Race* (Princeton, NJ: Princeton University Press, 1996).
17. Kwame A. Appiah, *The Ethics of Identity* (Princeton, NJ: Princeton University Press, 2005), and Kwame A. Appiah, "Toward a New Cosmopolitanism," *The New York Times Magazine,* January 1, 2006, sec. 6: 30–38, 52.

CONTRIBUTORS

Annette Dula, visiting scholar, University of Pittsburgh, Center for Bioethics and Health Law, and senior research associate at the Center for Values and Social Policy in the Philosophy Department at the University of Colorado, Boulder.

Kevin FitzGerald is senior research scholar in the Center for Clinical Bioethics at the Georgetown University Medical Center and is research associate professor in the Department of Oncology.

Jorge L. A. Garcia is professor of philosophy in the Department of Philosophy at Boston College and visiting professor in the Department of Linguistics and Philosophy, MIT.

Segun Gbadegesin is professor of philosophy in the Department of Philosophy at Howard University.

Ezra E. H. Griffith is professor of psychiatry and of African American studies at Yale University.

Patricia A. King is the Carmack Waterhouse Professor of Law, Medicine, Ethics, and Public Policy at Georgetown University Law Center, and adjunct professor in the Department of Health Policy and Management, School of Hygiene and Public Health at Johns Hopkins University.

Edmund D. Pellegrino is the chairman of the President's Council on Bioethics, and professor emeritus of medicine and medical ethics at the Center for Clinical Bioethics at Georgetown University Medical Center. He was the John Carroll Professor of Medicine and Medical Ethics and the former director of the Kennedy Institute of Ethics, the Center for Advanced Study of Ethics at Georgetown University, and the Center for Clinical Bioethics.

Reginald L. Peniston is the chief of surgery at the James A. Haley Veterans' Hospital in Tampa, Florida.

Lawrence J. Prograis Jr. is Senior Scientist for Special Programs and Bioethics in the Division of Allergy, Immunology, and Transplantation within the National Institute of Allergy and Infectious Diseases, National Institutes of Health, and affiliated scholar in the Center for Clinical Bioethics, Georgetown University.

Charmaine Royal is assistant professor in the Department of Pediatrics and Child Health (Division of Medical Genetics) and director of the GenEthics Unit in the National Human Genome Center at Howard University.

Cheryl J. Sanders is professor of Christian ethics in the School of Divinity at Howard University.

INDEX

Abu Ghraib prison, 105
affirmative action, 56, 75
African American, as term, 155–56
African American Heart Failure Trial
(A-HeFT) and BiDil, 11, 21n19, 22n30,
84–85, 137, 144–45
African American perspectives on culture
and biomedical ethics, ix–xxi, 1–23, 129;
and African traditional folkways, xvi–xvii;
antimajoritarian and antiutilitarian, 4;
antisituationist, 4, 5; benefits for contemporary thought, 6–8; and bioethics
discipline, x–xi, xii, xiii; and clinical
ethical decision making, xiv–xv, 127–36;
and cultural relativism, 2–3, 18–20n18;
defining culture, ix–x; and degraded
antilife bioethics, 8; development of the
current volume, xii–xv; elements that
ought to characterize, 4–5; and an "ethics
of trust," 4; ethnoracial issues, 12–15; and
families, 4; and Garcia's standpoint
epistemology, x, xiii, 3, 154, 156; and
human dignity, 4–5; humanizing influence
of, 7–8; implications for other cultural
groups, xv–xvii; and individualism, 5–6;
methodology of, 1, 2, 58–59; and moral
absolutism, xviii–xix; moral norms at
work in, 1, 2; moral philosophical
questions, xviii–xx; and moral relativism,
xviii–xix; and 1992 article/conference,
xi–xii, 4–6, 18–21n18; and patient
autonomy, 4; and political thought, 4, 6–7,
16n13, 17n14, 129–31; professional moral
obligations, xvi–xvii; the promise of, 1–3;
and racial concepts in medical research,
xv, 8–12, 137–51; and religious faith/
insights, xvii, 4, 6; and scientism, 4; and
sociopolitical concerns, xii–xiii; "standpoint
epistemology," x, xiii, 3, 154, 156; topics of,

1, 2; and unique moral claims, 1–2,
18–20n18; and virtue ethics, 3, 154.
See also personal narratives of African
American medical professionals
African traditional culture: concepts of
health, 95; folk healing and legacy of,
95–98; and moral weight of culture in
ethics, 26, 34, 35, 39–43; professional
moral obligations with regard to, xvi–xvii;
Yoruba customs, 26, 39–40, 42–43
Agency for Healthcare Research and Quality
(AHRQ), 73, 76
Alcoa, 56
Alexander v. Sandoval (2001), 78
American Cancer Society, 54, 60
American Enterprise Institute, 49, 55, 56, 59
*An American Health Dilemma: A Medical
History of African Americans and the
Problem of Race* (Byrd and Clayton), 99
American Journal of Public Health, 59
American Medical Association, 49–50
American Petroleum Institute, 56
American Psychological Association, 59
The Apostolic Faith (Azusa Street revival
newspaper), 97
Appelbaum, P. S., 118–21
Appiah, Anthony, 8, 155–56
asthma deaths, 48
Audi, Robert, 154
autonomy: and African American bioethical
perspectives, 4, 7–8; ethical issue of,
40–41
Avise, J. C., 140

Bad Blood (Jones), 52
Baldwin, James, 113
Ball, R. M., 140
Bamshad, M., 139–41
Banner, William Augustus, 132–35

Index

Index

gynecological experimentation, nineteenth century, 99–100

Hardimon, Michael, 9
Harlan, Justice John Marshall, 69
Harlem Renaissance, 107
The Health and Physique of the Negro American (Du Bois), 73, 81
health disparities: and American debate about race and equality, 72–75; asthma deaths, 48; drafts of National Healthcare Disparities Report (NHDR) (2003), 54–55, 76; federal and private efforts to address, 47–48, 73; and genomic medicine, 141–42; health status, 68; and individual patient responsibilities, 59–60, 77, 79; infant mortality rates, 48; Institute of Medicine (IOM) report (2002), 49–50, 57–58, 59, 69, 71, 73, 78–79; physicians' views, 75–76; transracial disparities, 12–13. *See also* health disparities and deliberate deceptions; race, equality, and health policy
health disparities and deliberate deceptions, xiv, 47–65; corporate-sponsored think tanks, 47–48, 55–56, 60–61; corporations' vested interests and deceptive assertions, 48, 55–61; deceptions regarding HHS's 2003 National Healthcare Disparities Report (NHDR), 54–55; deceptions regarding Tuskegee Syphilis Study, 51–53; environmental pollutants/toxins and health, 50–51; and federal/private efforts to address health disparities, 47–48; and flawed research methodology, 58–59; individual spokespeople for conservative think tanks, 60–61; and personal responsibility issue, 59–60; and physician race bias/negative stereotyping, 49–50, 57–58, 61; smoking issue, 51, 53–54, 58, 59, 60–61; stories that whitewash health disparities/dismiss role of race, 49–55
Healthy People 2010, 61–62
Heller, John, 100
Herder, Johann Gottfried von, 28

Heritage Foundation, 55, 56, 59
Herrnstein, Richard J., 59
Higginbotham, Leon, 113, 114
Holiness-Pentecostal tradition, 97–98
Howard University conference on African American perspectives on bioethics (1992), xi
Howard University Hospital (HUH), 135
Human Genome Project (HGP), 75, 82–83, 138, 139, 141
Hurricane Katrina, 80

immigrant groups, xv
Incidents in the Life of a Slave Girl (Brent), 112
inclusion requirements for NIH-funded research, 82, 86
infant mortality rates, 48, 80
informed consent, 39–40
Institute of Medicine (IOM) report on disparities in health care (2002), 49–50, 57–58, 59, 69, 71, 73, 78–79, 143; and physician bias, 57; and research methods, 58
Institutional Review Boards (IRBs), 53
Iraq, U.S.-led invasion of, 129–30
I've Known Rivers (Lawrence-Lightfoot), 116

Jackson, Jesse, 113
Johnson, Carolyn, 21n19, 137, 148
Johnson, President Lyndon B., 70
Jones, James, 52
Jonsen, Albert, 1, 154–55, 157n11
Journal of the American Medical Association, 59, 60–61

Kahn, Jonathan, 21n19
Kaiser Foundation, 47–48, 57
Kant, Immanuel, 7
Kass, Leon, 17n15
Keita, O. Y., 140–41, 146–47
Kellogg Foundation, 47–48
Keyes, Alan, 130
kidney transplantation allocation policies, 71
King, Martin Luther, Jr., 113

Index